foodist

foodist

Using Real Food and Real Science
to Lose Weight Without Dieting

Darya Pino Rose

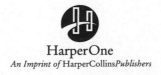

HarperOne
An Imprint of HarperCollins*Publishers*

HarperOne

This book is written as a source of information only. The information contained in this book should by no means be considered a substitute for the advice of a qualified medical professional, who should always be consulted before beginning any new diet, exercise, or other health program.

FIRST EDITION

Designed by Kris Tobiassen

Library of Congress Cataloging-in-Publication Data

Rose, Darya Pino.
    Foodist : using real food and real science to lose weight without dieting / by Darya Pino Rose. — First edition.
        pages cm
    ISBN 978–0–06–220125–6
    1. Nutrition. 2. Weight loss. 3. Food—Psychological aspects. I. Title.
    RA784.R649 2013
    613.2—dc23   2012046666

13 14 15 16 17 RRD(H) 10 9 8 7 6 5 4 3 2 1

To my dad, for believing in me since before I was born.

CONTENTS

PART III: THE DAILY FOODIST

PART I

HEALTHSTYLE

"We are what we repeatedly do. Excellence, then, is not an act, but a habit."

—ARISTOTLE

ONE

"DIET" IS A FOUR-LETTER WORD

What This Book Is, and Isn't

"I've been on a diet for two weeks and all I've lost is two weeks."
—TOTIE FIELDS, COMEDIAN

"I don't like stuff that sucks."
—*BEAVIS AND BUTTHEAD*

"Life itself is the proper binge."
—JULIA CHILD

Dieters are a funny breed and by many criteria could be classified as insane. Gleefully participate in self-inflicted suffering? Check. Restrict entire categories of edible, nutritious, and tasty food? Check. Do the same thing over and over again and expect different results? Check. Throw in a couple of face tattoos and straitjackets, and we'll be ready for the asylum.

Amazingly, there are very few of us who do not belong to the dieter tribe. Dieting, and specifically chronic dieting (bouncing back and forth between various diets, food philosophies, and, ahem, body sizes), is a popular hobby in the twenty-first century. A combination of supersizing and unrealistic beauty standards has forced most of us to question the way we eat and look, and the dieting industry has been more than happy to offer us thousands of weight-loss solutions every year. Bless their hearts.

I would say it is unfortunate that their pills, programs, and bonus DVDs haven't really worked out, but now that I'm a foodist, I see the failure of the dieting industry to make us thinner or healthier as one of the luckiest mess-ups of our generation. Just imagine if it worked. How horrible would it be if, in order to look and feel amazing, you had to deprive yourself of foods you love for the rest of your life, skipping birthday cake and Michelin-rated restaurants, just so you can feel good about yourself when you look in the mirror? Seriously, screw that. It isn't necessary, even if you did have the willpower to pull it off (and you probably don't). There is a better way, and all it takes is thinking about food, health, and weight loss not like a dieter, but like a foodist.

If you've tried any weight-loss program in the past, you probably know from experience that dieters almost never eat food. Sure, dieters eat protein, fat, carbs (though they may try not to), calories, calcium, and omega-3s, but to them food is just a vehicle to ingest essential nutrients, not the ultimate reason for eating. I know this because I was a chronic dieter for most of my life, and over almost two decades I've tried nearly every weight-loss strategy under the sun.

My dieting adventure started unintentionally. One sunny morning in sixth grade I walked into the kitchen to find my mother making what looked like a milkshake. Thinking I might have won the break-fast lottery, I enthusiastically inquired what it was. She explained that it was indeed a chocolate shake, but it was for a new diet that was sup-posed to help her lose weight. My eleven-year-old translation: we can have chocolate milkshakes for breakfast and not worry about getting fat. My mom agreed to share, and breakfast was never the same again.

Over the next few years I went from SlimFast every morning to a diet almost completely free of fat (remember the 1990s?). By the time I got to college, it was nothing but meat, eggs, and cottage cheese according to Dr. Atkins. From there I moved to *The South Beach Diet* and started running marathons to burn extra calories. In other words, I was the perfect example of what Michael Pollan, author of *The Omnivore's Dilemma* and real-food hero, aptly describes as our "national eating disorder."[1] I embraced every new diet as if it had the potential to solve all my problems, following every ridiculous rule without question or exception.

In retrospect the most interesting part is not that I tried all these diets (clearly I was not alone in my efforts), but that I was good at them. I was very thin (i.e., "successful") on my low-fat regimen in high school—I was a ballerina and definitely looked the part. After I stopped dancing and put some weight back on, I had no trouble abandoning bread, rice, and potatoes for several years while I got back down to size 0 on the Atkins diet. I gladly woke up at 5:00 A.M. for two-hour workouts every weekday and clocked three-hour-long runs every Sunday for marathon training during my first few years of graduate school. Though my successes may have been fleeting, a weak will has never been the reason. The problem wasn't me. The problem was that starving yourself of energy, nutrients, and pleasure is not the most effective way to attain—let alone *maintain*—the body you want. It is also no way to live your life.

Chronic dieters believe that success comes from sacrifice. If only we could deprive ourselves a little more, punish our bodies even harder, then we could finally look amazing and, of course, be happy. But as someone who has tortured herself in every way imaginable, I can guarantee you that this path does not lead to happiness. Why? Because it turns life into a constant struggle. You never really win if you're dieting. When you are constantly depriving yourself, happiness is always just out of reach. So even if you could confidently identify the best, most effective restrictive diet, why should this be your goal? Shouldn't there be more to life than constantly denying yourself the things you enjoy? Now you're thinking like a foodist.

As simple and logical as this sounds, I know from experience that ending deprivation is tough for chronic dieters. "No pain, no gain" is fundamental to our psyche—don't we deserve to suffer for being so fat? Most of us have been victims of a vicious, convoluted feedback loop through which we are rewarded for our sacrifices with temporary (but often dramatic) weight loss at the beginning of each new diet. This creates the illusion of success. But you have to ask yourself: shouldn't *real* success be defined as lasting—not temporary—weight loss?

Nutritionists and M.D.s haven't helped much either. Virtually all weight-loss experts tell us we need to eat less and move more to lose weight, with the obvious implication being that we need to diet (deprive ourselves) and exercise (suffer at the gym) to achieve our goals. You can't break the first law of thermodynamics—it's science! But this line of thinking neglects the reasons we are compelled to overeat in the first place and doesn't give us the tools we need to actually implement their simple "eat less, move more, lose weight" equation. It also implies that failure stems from a lack of willpower (why aren't you eating less, like you're supposed to?), rather than from a plan that fails to account for the nuances of the human psyche. How many people do you know who eat solely for fuel? All the thin people, right? Not a chance. Sure, we all sometimes eat because we're hungry. But the specific foods we choose and how much we eat are largely influenced by our habits and environment. In other words, it is not the concept of eating less to lose weight that is wrong, but the idea that we can lose weight and keep it off without accounting for why we make the choices we do.

My own experiences convinced me that willpower was not the missing piece of the equation. After all, I was following all the rules, but maintaining my weight was still a constant struggle. At the time I didn't know what I was missing, but I was confident that humans have not always had this problem and that something about the current weight-loss paradigm must be wrong. It wasn't until my second year of grad school that I realized I finally had enough training in biology to go directly to the scientific literature for answers. Before, I had relied on diet books and magazine articles to fumble my way through different weight-loss strategies. Now that I had the knowledge and lab experience to read and understand the science, I wanted to see the data for myself.

Not surprisingly, even at this stage I went about my research all wrong. From my chronic dieter's perspective I was looking for the perfect diet, partially expecting some version of low-carb to be the answer (this had been the easiest, after all). So in the beginning my findings were very discouraging. The first thing I learned is that for the most part, diets don't work for long-term weight loss. In fact, going on some sort of weight-loss diet is actually a significant predictor of *weight gain*.[2] D'oh. That said, you can lose weight, at least for a little while, on any diet. Compared to low-fat diets, low-carb diets tend to have a more dramatic effect on weight loss in the beginning, but the weight will usually creep back on within a year. Five percent of the population does manage to keep weight off permanently after dieting, but the method they use to get there doesn't seem to matter. These people have somehow managed to integrate healthier habits into their lives and make permanent lifestyle changes.

What about people who are naturally thin or never get fat—what do they eat? Once again the data show that macronutrient (carb, fat, and protein) ratios have little impact on whether a person or population becomes overweight. People can thrive on low-fat diets, high-fat diets, low-carb diets, and low-protein diets. As Michael Pollan explores in his book *In Defense of Food,* the most consistent predictor of weight gain and poor health is how much processed food people eat.[3] Whether it's low-fat or low-carb, industrially processed foods are more likely to hinder rather than help with weight control.

But *what* you eat is only one part of the equation. *How* and even *why* you eat also have a significant impact on your long-term health and body weight. Habits such as chewing thoroughly and eating slowly are more common among normal-weight than overweight individuals. Cultures that encourage eating for enjoyment (e.g., the French) and health (e.g., Okinawans) have a lower incidence of obesity than other industrial societies. In other words, the science tells us that it is more important to focus on habits and overall healthy eating patterns rather than carbs and protein. Moreover, psychology and food culture can be as crucial as the types of foods you eat in determining your long-term success.

When I first realized the implications of the science, I hesitated. You mean I should try to be healthy instead of skinny? I should give up my protein bars? I should eat breakfast? I can eat carbs?! And, strangest of all, I should *stop* dieting? I didn't see how any of these things could do anything but make me gain weight. But I trusted science more than *Cosmo,* or even *Shape* magazine, and decided to give it a try. I figured if it didn't work after a couple of weeks, I could go back to my cabbage soup and grapefruit and get back on track. So I took a deep breath, stopped counting calories, and started eating food. Real food. And for the first time in my life, I lost weight effortlessly.

The first changes I made were pretty simple. I *added* regular breakfast, intact and whole grains (the difference will be clear soon), and seasonal produce from the farmers market. I also included more legumes like beans and lentils. I stopped drinking diet soda and eating energy bars and other diet foods artificially high in protein and fiber. I also cut my cardio workouts down to thirty minutes (from sixty-plus minutes) and focused more on strength training and free weights. Not only did I lose weight when I incorporated these changes, but the proportions and shape of my body transformed into what I was striving for all along: one that was more slender and toned, rather than muscly with trouble spots (don't worry, boys, because you have more testosterone, becoming a foodist can also help you build muscles).

I also lost the cravings for sweets and heavy foods that I'd struggled with my entire life. Even on the various low-carb diets I tried, I longed for bran muffins and chocolate. Since I've started eating real food, sugar cravings no longer haunt me, and I enjoy desserts whenever I feel like it, which is far less often. Managing my portions is much easier. Meals are satisfying, and I am hungry at the appropriate times. The stress and anxiety I used to feel about food and my weight have completely disappeared.

But that's not even the best part of the story. Something else happened when I made that tentative commitment to focus on health instead of weight loss. After years of battling and sometimes even hating food, I discovered I loved it. I had recently moved from Berkeley to San Francisco, and some friends introduced me to the food scene. Until then I thought I knew what good food tasted like, but I was completely unprepared for the experience I had during my first truly spectacular meal. In San Francisco, ingredients shine. Yes, the chefs are innovative and brilliant, but what differentiated this food from anything I'd had in the past is the simple idea that excellent food starts with excellent ingredients. San Francisco opened my eyes to what was possible in the culinary world and, amazingly, it is based on the same principles that freed me from dieting tyranny.

Before this time I had assumed, like most people, that healthy food tasted bad, or at least worse than anything people would actually want to eat. Of course, when you're told rice cakes and protein bars are "healthy," then this is true. It is even true of the soggy frozen spinach and mealy pink tomatoes that passed for vegetables when I was growing up. But just like delicious San Francisco food, the healthiest food is made from high-quality, peak-of-the-season ingredients grown with care by people who are passionate about their product. I had always thought a carrot was a carrot or a chicken was a chicken, but this couldn't be farther from the truth.

Weather and soil quality are the biggest determinants of the nutritional value of agricultural products (including the animals that feed on the plants). They are also the most important factors in how food tastes. A tomato from your garden in the summer tastes worlds better than one from the supermarket in January, and the same rules of seasonality apply to broccoli and even meat. It makes sense when you think about it. Isn't the quality of every product ultimately determined by the quality of its starting materials? What's amazing is that this fact transforms healthy food from something unappealing into something delicious. Fortunately for me and my grad-student budget, I could get the same ingredients used by fancy San Francisco restaurants at the local farmers market for a fraction of the price. Once I made this discovery, I could never go back to mediocre food.

It is difficult to quantify the impact of loving food instead of fighting it. Eating healthy becomes a joy, so weight loss comes naturally. Friends look at your meals with envy instead of pity. Your goals transform from burdens into fun new projects. Psychologically, one of the most important aspects of your life—the food you eat three times a day and the meals you share with friends and family—pulls a complete one-eighty and changes from stressful and difficult to joyful and delicious. The old way of dieting, and the suffering it brings, suddenly seem so unnecessary.

Foodists do not diet. Modern weight-loss diets are temporary eating plans that emphasize single nutrients and restriction over real food and lifelong habits. Foodists, in contrast, focus on real, high-quality foods in order to optimize our quality of life. We understand that how you look and feel about your body is important, but that true happiness also comes from excellent health, a fulfilling social life, rich cultural experiences, and physical enjoyment. Don't get me wrong, my goal is to help you lose weight. But I want to make sure your success is permanent and that you don't suffer in the process. Popular weight-loss diets sacrifice all the other aspects of life and happiness for the sake of dropping weight rapidly. But foodists know that being thinner does not solve all your problems, and if you neglect the rest of your life to get there, the weight will find its way back. As a foodist, I want more than a perfect body; I want an amazing life.

For these reasons my philosophy on food has nothing to do fat, carbs, or calories. I approach food and health with only one unshakable belief: that life should be awesome. What you eat should always enhance, and never detract from, your quality of life. You should be able to look and feel your best not just while starving yourself for a few weeks or months, but for as long as you care enough to try. Your food should taste delicious, whether it's healthy or not, and you should never feel guilty for what you choose.

Foodist is a training manual to make real food, and therefore real, lasting weight control, a permanent part of your life. Knowing what to eat isn't the toughest part of losing weight. There are thin, healthy people everywhere along the diet spectrum, and most of us already know that broccoli is a better choice than cheesecake. What's difficult is navigating a world that constantly steers us away from better food and better health. The challenge is actually *doing* what we know is best.

Foodist will teach you how to overcome the daily obstacles and ingrained habits that prevent you from reaching your goals. Since we all face different challenges, it will also help you tailor your strategies for your own lifestyle and preferences, making sure the path you choose will work for you in the long term. You'll learn the basics of both nutrition and psychology, so you understand not just what to eat, but also when, where, why, and how to choose foods that optimize your health and happiness. Our goal isn't just weight loss. We want to make sure the effort you put in now gets you where you want to be, but more important is that it helps you stay there.

This book is divided into three parts. In Part I, I aim to convince you once and for all that dieting is a fool's mission that in the long run does more harm than good. This is not bad news, though, because I then present a more effective (and vastly more enjoyable) alternative: building rewarding habits. Habits make eating healthy even easier than eating unhealthy, since they are automatic behaviors that do not require willpower. Built into this approach are joy and pleasure, since it is impossible for new habits to form without an associated reward. If healthy eating isn't fun, it isn't going to work.

Focusing on real food instead of those specialty, highly processed diet foods is the secret to making healthy food enjoyable. My recipe for how to make cauliflower taste as good as french fries (p. 237) has convinced hundreds of skeptics that vegetables aren't just palatable, but can be insanely delicious. There will always be excuses to eat unhealthy foods (and these are never off-limits), but as a foodist you'll have just as many delicious reasons to eat real, healthy foods. Not only do they make your taste buds happy, but unlike processed foods they'll make you feel great and fit into your clothes after eating them. For dieters and nondieters alike, this is a game changer.

Yet as simple as it sounds, eating real food is not always straightforward. After writing multiple books and hundreds of pages explaining what it means to eat healthy, Michael Pollan still has readers clamoring for more details on how to do it. When I asked him why he thinks people continue to struggle with this, he offered two reasons. "The message 'Eat real food' is all but drowned out by $30-plus billion in marketing messages from the food industry. Think about the supermarket: the fresh produce is silent while the cereal aisle is full of screamers. The message gets lost," Pollan told me. We grew up learning to pay attention to nutrients, not foods, and in the process humble whole foods were virtually eliminated from our regular eating habits.

A second issue is that eating real food requires a skill set few of us ever acquired. As a result, finding, preparing, and even identifying real food can be a challenge. "Real food is not as convenient as the other stuff, which has been engineered for ease of use, not to mention addictiveness and a long shelf life," says Pollan. "This puts real food at a real disadvantage."

Part II confronts these issues head-on by giving you a blueprint to get started. This includes analyzing your own diet to understand which of your habits you should target to make the biggest impact on your health and body weight. These will be different for everyone, and I'll take you through the process of identifying and modifying your habits in a way that is best for your lifestyle. Part II teaches you how to set up your kitchen, living, and work environments as well, so that you're never lacking in healthy, delicious options. This section also goes beyond food choices, highlighting the peripheral but equally important habits that impact your health and weight, including eating slowly and mindfully and being active instead of sedentary.

Last, Part II contains a detailed troubleshooting section and explores the most fundamental difference between a foodist and a chronic dieter: lifelong weight control. There is an art and science to being a foodist that includes having an intimate understanding of what it takes for your life to be awesome and also adjusting to life's inevitable changes. Maintaining your weight requires ongoing self-experimentation as you shape and adjust your core habits to the evolving demands of your life. Part II teaches you these skills and also offers a recalibration plan in case you get stuck along the way.

Part III walks you through the nitty-gritty of daily living, showing you how to make the best food decisions at home, at work, in restaurants, and while traveling. It includes tips for taming a family of picky eaters and how to subtly deflect attention from your healthier choices in situations where virtuous behavior isn't welcome. These can be as straightforward as changing the language you use to describe and think about food (e.g., kale is "tasty," not "healthy") or dimming the lights to help you and your dining partners eat slower. Tricks like these are invaluable, because each one removes a barrier that keeps you from your goals and sets you up for long-term success. The book closes on a philosophical note, explaining why food matters and why you'll be happier and have greater success if you care about yours.

If you picked up this book, there's a good chance this is not the first time you hoped a new eating plan would help you lose weight. But even if you've never tried to diet in the past, *Foodist* can help you achieve your goals. I will give you the tools you need to manage all aspects of your health for the long haul. Not only will you permanently build better habits into your daily life; you'll also enjoy the food you eat more than you ever thought possible.

Food shouldn't be about sacrifice. It should enrich your life by satisfying your palate, making you fit and healthy, and bringing you closer to your family, friends, and community. For most of human existence this was the case, but in the last hundred years or so we've shifted to viewing food as more of a vehicle to achieve our goals rather than an end in itself. We treat food as a weight-loss tool, a source of nutrients, a sinful indulgence, or an excuse to procrastinate rather than something that has value for its own sake. I wrote *Foodist* to turn our attention back to real food as something essential to our happiness, as something that makes life awesome.

TWO

THE MYTH OF WILLPOWER

You Don't Fail Diets—They Fail You

"It is a hard matter, my fellow citizens, to argue
with the belly, since it has no ears."

—CATO THE ELDER

"To promise not to do a thing is the surest way in the world to
make a body want to go and do that very thing."

—MARK TWAIN

I know how difficult it can be for a dieter to stop looking for a quick fix, even when our better judgment tells us that restriction diets will only help us keep weight off for a limited period of time. It's still incredibly tempting to put on your superhero outfit with the big *S* for Self-Control on the chest. You've conquered your hunger in the past and lost that twenty-plus pounds. Why not just do it again for a couple of months? Once you hit your goal weight, then you can start with this whole healthy eating thing for maintenance.

I know it's tempting. But I hope this chapter will convince you that the belief that you can will yourself thin actually does you more harm than good, that instead of getting you closer to where you want to be, it just causes you to waste time that could be used to develop the habits needed to achieve your goals *and stay there*. Restrictive dieting and excessive workouts won't get you ahead faster. They actually do the opposite, holding you back both physically and mentally from better health and happiness.

THE WEAKNESS OF WILLPOWER

Does stronger willpower lead to greater and longer-lasting weight loss? Let's tackle this question head-on, because the answer will help us find a better path. My own story suggests that there is more to weight loss than willpower, since it wasn't until I *stopped* trying to eat less that my weight came down easily. But the science shows that even the "successes"* I had on restriction diets are not typical.

Self-control has always been easy for me, but this isn't the case for most people, particularly when it comes to food. In their excellent book *Willpower: Rediscovering the Greatest Human Strength,* Roy Baumeister and John Tierney argue that humans can invoke incredible acts of will in certain circumstances,[1] but concede that dieting is a special case. Baumeister calls it "the Oprah Paradox," named for the popular TV personality and one of the most successful human beings on the planet, Oprah Winfrey. "Even people with excellent self-control can have a hard time consistently controlling their weight."[2]

Despite Winfrey's obvious personal capabilities and limitless resources, her weight struggles have been notoriously rocky. Anyone who

---

*I use quotes with the word "success" as it relates to diets, because I don't think being miserable should count as success. But dieting success is typically defined by weight loss, not happiness, and that I definitely achieved.

has repeatedly tried and failed to maintain significant weight loss can sympathize with her plight. If you are accustomed to being successful in other parts of your life, this dose of reality is particularly hard to swallow. We've been able to excel in so many different endeavors—why can't we just suck it up and get our weight under control? Indeed, Baumeister's research shows that people with more willpower typically have better success at school, in business, and in their personal lives than people with less self-control, but the difference is much less pronounced in controlling body weight, at least in the long term. Although more willpower does help people stick to their diets and therefore lose more weight temporarily, over the course of their lives the strong-willed only weigh slightly less than the weak-willed.

One reason for this is that willpower is dependent on blood sugar.[3] Like a muscle, willpower has limited capacity, and when exercised extensively it can become depleted. Also like a muscle, the primary fuel your brain uses to exert willpower is sugar from your blood. So when your blood sugar is low (i.e., when you're hungry, which when you're dieting is pretty much all the time), your willpower is weaker than ever, and the only way to fix it is to eat. You can see the difficulty this can cause when you're making food decisions. Throwing exercise into the equation—something dieters use to intentionally burn more calories (i.e., use more blood sugar)—only makes things more problematic. Baumeister and Tierney call it a nutritional catch-22: the less you eat and the more you exercise, the less likely you will be to make good food decisions down the stretch and maintain your weight loss.

The blood-sugar issue also makes it more difficult for people who are already metabolically compromised. If you are overweight or have a history of poor eating habits, then there's an excellent chance you have developed or are on your way to developing metabolic syndrome. *Metabolic syndrome* is a series of health problems that stem from poor blood-sugar control and lead to increased risk for heart disease, stroke, and type 2 diabetes. The main symptoms are increased body fat around the midsection and insulin resistance. When people lose sensitivity to insulin, they have difficulty maintaining stable blood-sugar (glucose) levels and are subject to large blood-glucose swings in response to food intake. Since willpower is sensitive to these shifting glucose levels, metabolic syndrome makes it even harder to maintain your willpower and control your eating throughout the course of the day.

To make matters worse, hunger and exercise are not the only ways to deplete willpower. Research by Baumeister and other scientists has shown that we only have a single stock of willpower for everything we do, and any task that requires self-control will deplete your resolve in challenges that seem otherwise unrelated. For instance, if you spend a good portion of your afternoon trying to restrain yourself from decapitating a particularly obnoxious client, you're more likely to give in to temptation and order from your favorite pizza joint rather than stop at Whole Foods to pick up organic vegetables and fish for dinner, as you had planned. Inadequate sleep is another factor that diminishes willpower by depleting blood-sugar reserves, and sleep-deprived people are more likely to be impulsive and make bad decisions than their well-rested peers. Women experiencing PMS, as you might expect, are also depleted in the self-control department, as are most parents of small children.

Food and eating are often the first places we slip when our wills are weakened. We tend to put our professional and family responsibilities ahead of our personal health when prioritizing our daily actions, so when our mental resources are being taxed, our food choices feel like a trivial sacrifice. One reason for this is that the consequences are not immediately apparent; they accumulate over weeks, months, and years—too slow for us to notice in our daily lives. Another reason we give in to food temptations more readily than to other desires is that subconsciously our brains are craving that hit of glucose, and we know that a handful of cookies or a bag of chips is the fastest way to make that happen. So unless you're confident you'll never again have to wake up a little earlier than you'd prefer or need to control yourself in any other part of your life, you probably shouldn't rely on willpower to see you through your long-term diet goals.

DIETING MAKES IT WORSE

The biological reasons I just described explaining why willpower is unreliable for controlling your weight are depressing enough. But for chronic dieters, the story gets even sadder. Although all of us are subject to willpower lapses as a result of blood-sugar depletion, dieters are a special group whose restrictive goals make them more likely than nondieters to dramatically overdo it in the face of culinary temptations. To put it bluntly, dieting makes it worse.

Unlike normal eaters, dieters give themselves a daily allowance for calories (or carbs, or fat—pick your poison), below which they are virtuous and above which they have failed (at least for the day). The problem is that this self-imposed boundary gives rise to a phenomenon that scientists refer to as *counterregulatory eating*, also known as the "what-the-hell effect." Researchers have shown that once dieters cross the allowance they have set for themselves, they chock up the day as a failure and rationalize any additional overindulgence with, "Oh what the hell. I've already screwed up the day. I might as well enjoy it now." The problem is that once dieters reach this point, they stop paying attention and ultimately eat far more than nondieters would in the same situation. Even more dangerous is the fact that, although dieters know they didn't stick to their goals for the day, most are completely clueless about how much they actually consumed during the lapse. They don't realize that these episodes can undo days and even weeks of restricted eating, ultimately causing weight gain rather than loss.

The reason dieters are prone to this behavior is that restricted eating teaches you to ignore your internal satiety cues, the biological signals that tell us if we are hungry or full. For example, if you are hungry, but the diet you are following says you can't eat for another two hours, you force yourself to ignore the pangs and power through. Not only does this deplete your willpower and make it more likely you'll break your diet later in the day; it also teaches your brain not to listen to your body. This is a double-edged sword, however, because it doesn't just train you to ignore hunger. Not paying attention to satiety signals also means you can't tell when you're full, which can cause you to eat far more than your body actually desires.

Without internal guidance cues, dieters depend more on external signals for when to start and stop eating. Relying on external eating cues means you are more likely to eat just because food is available and finish everything on your plate regardless of its size or your hunger level. You're also more likely to eat until you've polished off an entire bag of chips, the episode of *Breaking Bad* you're watching ends, or it is physically impossible to shove another bite down your throat without exploding. Needless to say, this sort of behavior is not a recipe for long-term weight control.

Ignoring internal satiety cues has other implications as well. With today's information overload and the disintegration of traditional food cultures that have historically dictated when, where, and how much is appropriate to eat, we are bombarded with cues that trigger us to want to consume more food more often. Food packages have been transformed into easily transportable containers meant for eating on the go. Supersizing and buffets are considered good deals, not unbridled gluttony. TV commercials encourage us to embrace a "fourth meal," hoping we won't notice the hundreds of extra calories per day. Snacking at your desk or in front of the TV isn't just normal; it's expected. This environment is hard for even nondieters to navigate without experiencing significant weight gain. But for dieters, who have trouble telling when they're hungry and when they're full, all these eating triggers add an extra level of difficulty.

Resisting "eat now" and "eat more" triggers all day long creates more opportunities for our willpower to break down and increases the likelihood that we'll overeat. Moreover, even if we could rely on our internal satiety cues, since we're dieting our bodies would likely be telling us that we are in fact hungry and that popcorn is sounding pretty darn good about now. When every food choice you confront becomes a difficult decision, your willpower is constantly being depleted, even during choices that nondieters wouldn't think twice about. As a result, dieting makes weight loss even harder than it needs to be.

IF YOU'VE GOT IT, DON'T USE IT

You might be wondering at this point if weight loss is even possible. If we need to eat less to lose weight, but eating less makes weight loss impossible, how in the name of skinny jeans are we supposed to drop those extra pounds?

The answer may at first seem counterintuitive. Since willpower cannot be relied upon to help us make the right food choices, our best bet is to not use it. At least not constantly, the way dieters try to. Baumeister and Tierney explain: "We've said that willpower is humans' greatest strength, but the best strategy is not to rely on it in all situations. Save it for emergencies."[4] This is their conclusion after Baumeister and others completed a study that combined the results of many experiments (a meta-analysis) that measured willpower. The surprising finding was that people who had the highest measures of self-control seemed to use it the least. Instead, they focused their efforts on establishing automatic behaviors, or habits, ultimately reducing their need for effortful self-control.[5]

Treating long-term repetitive behaviors like eating and exercising as individual acts that require willpower in every instance creates many opportunities for failure. The more effective strategy is to use willpower to set up routines that eventually become automatic. When these behaviors become habitual and no longer require mental effort, willpower is reserved for the most critical decisions. As the researchers conclude

9 Surefire Ways to Sabotage Your Weight Loss

1. Rely on willpower

Even if you're one of those people with an iron will, no one can hold out forever. Willpower is notoriously unreliable, and if you're ever sleepy, hungry, tipsy, grumpy, sad, happy, lazy, or all of the above, your weakness will eventually win.

2. Forget the difference between temporary and permanent

Is your goal to fit into a size 4? Almost anyone can get there by following a strict enough diet and workout regimen for a set amount of time. The question is, how long do you want to stay there? If your goals are intended to be permanent, your dietary and fitness modifications need to be as well.

3. Start a really hard workout regimen

Having someone kick your ass in boot camp may sound like what you need to get in shape, but how long do you really think you will subject yourself to pain and suffering before you give up on exercise completely? Most people don't last two months.

4. Never learn to eat mindfully

One of the biggest differences between American culture and those of less obese nations (e.g., France) is our complete and utter lack of food culture. In healthier cultures, mealtime is an important event when people gather to share good food and stories from the day. With these habits come standards for portion sizes, eating speed, and nutritional balance.

Sadly, it's unlikely the United States will suddenly establish a healthy food culture in time to help the majority of the population. But you can get a lot of the benefits yourself by learning to eat mindfully (see chapter 7). Mindful eating helps you slow down, savor your food, and appreciate each bite. For these reasons it is incredibly effective at helping with portion control—without leaving you feeling deprived.

In our culture, mindful eating is very difficult and takes some practice. It's hard to slow down when your friends are wolfing down food by the handful. But it is possible. Practice when you're alone, and it will be easier when you're with friends.

5. Ignore how much you miss your favorite foods

Love ice cream? Can you go your entire life without it? What about six months? Or do you just plan to hold out as long as you can before the next inevitable binge? Cold turkey isn't necessary if you develop a healthy relationship with your favorite treats.

6. Assume that what worked for someone else will work for you

Have a friend who lost a ton of weight on the Atkins diet? Me too. I also have friends who lost weight doing the Master Cleanse or going vegan. Typically only the ones who make permanent habit changes can maintain it, so a plan that works for someone else will only work for you if you enjoy it and can incorporate it into your life. Everyone is different.

7. Dramatically restrict your eating

Starving is not fun. Nor are cravings. Nor is malnutrition. Limiting your calories to unrealistic lows is a great way to begin the cycle of yo-yo dieting that we all know and love. Enjoy!

8. Don't find deeper purpose in what and why you eat

This one may sound a bit esoteric, but bear with me. If the goal is to build healthy habits (which it should be), the people who have the most success are those who want to achieve more than a change in their appearance. Vegans believe so deeply that harming animals is wrong that they never stray from their diets. Locavores want to know and trace the source of all their foods. For some people, being told they will die if they do not change their habits is enough.

For myself, it's good to know that my habits are healthy and effective, but I've come to understand that how I eat is a way of life that has a deeper political, philosophical, and environmental impact than I ever imagined. It's also super tasty. For inspiration, check out the film *Food, Inc.* or read *The Omnivore's Dilemma,* by Michael Pollan.[6] You won't regret it.

9. Pick a diet that is super inconvenient

We all have our limits on how far we'll go to stick to an eating plan. Be sure to know yours. If you're too busy (or have too many taste buds) to eat a specific combination of foods every three hours—I know I couldn't—then don't pretend you can. Pick dietary changes you can handle; the little things do add up if you can maintain them for the long haul.

in the meta-analysis, "The main value of self-control may lie more in creating the healthy habit than in regulating behavior each day anew."[7]

Baumeister and Tierney's findings match precisely with my personal experiences in dieting. In the past when I attempted to lose weight by restricting my eating, limiting food was never difficult in the beginning—I was well-trained at overriding my hunger signals. But over time I would grow tired and look for new, less painful ways to achieve the same results. Since these hacks never worked out in the long term, I would eventually abandon the diet for a more promising one. Between diets or while I was on a diet that restricted certain food groups but not others (my favorite example is Atkins, with its unlimited-bacon breakfast), I had absolutely no control over my appetite and could put down quantities of food that would make an NFL lineman blush. Now that I have the habit of eating healthy food in reasonable quantities, it feels like the easiest, and at times the most indulgent, thing in the world. I tell people with pride that I eat whatever I want, but the reality is that I now want healthy food most of the time. Since my cravings are gone, I can eat dessert whenever I feel like it, but I only get the urge about once a week, sometimes less. My meals are also a fraction of the size they used to be, and I have trouble comprehending how I was ever able to eat such colossal quantities of food.

I still use willpower occasionally to control my eating. For example, if I have dinner reservations immediately following a workout, it takes some effort to not inhale the entire bread basket before my entree arrives. But for the most part healthy choices now come naturally to me, and the pain that comes from using my willpower and denying myself the things I want is no longer a daily occurrence. To put it another way, it is not just my body that has changed since I became a foodist; the way I think and feel about food is now fundamentally different.

Relying on willpower to get and keep you looking your best is not a winning strategy, but willpower does have a place in a foodist's life. Instead of squandering precious self-control on restrictive dieting, a foodist uses it to start building better habits. It's not hard to upgrade your healthstyle by eating all the delicious seasonal food that replaces the dimensionless processed stuff you grew up on. That's the fun part. What's tough is remembering to go to the farmers market or the grocery store regularly, so you have healthy food in your house and don't have an excuse to grab takeout for dinner, or teaching yourself to chew your food thoroughly when you're used to wolfing it down like a savage beast, or finding the time to make physical activity part of your day when you have a thousand and one things to do before noon. I'll teach you to use the willpower you have to build these kinds of habits into your life. Once they are automated, healthy choices come naturally and in many cases become even easier than your old ways. Then you can use your willpower for simpler, more manageable tasks, like that restaurant bread basket.

IT'S TIME TO GO ALL IN

Breaking your reliance on willpower requires giving up restrictive diets—and that means forever. Remember, dieting teaches you to ignore internal satiety signals and leaves you with nothing but external cues to tell you when to start and stop eating. These triggers require willpower to resist, and with every act of self-denial (and every drop in blood sugar) your resolve is weakened. The data consistently show that over time dieting is more likely to result in weight gain rather than weight loss. Dieting also makes your life suck, and that is unacceptable.

If you accept this premise that dieting is a bad idea, then you're ready to become a foodist. But the fact that you won't be relying as heavily on willpower doesn't mean your journey is going to be easy. It is important to keep in mind that, when you begin on a path toward healthier eating, you are going to face some obstacles. Habits take time to break and rebuild, and there are too many temptations and ways for your plans to be derailed to expect perfection from yourself. Deviations from your ideal will happen, so the best strategy is to plan for them, so you have more control. What's essential is that you do not let one unexpected slipup demolish your resolve. Being healthy isn't a destination; it's a journey. What works for you will change as your life commitments and circumstances evolve, so you must adapt and continue to experiment on yourself. It is also critical to understand that, for this strategy to be effective, you must adopt the long view and commit to becoming a healthy person no matter what setbacks come up along the way. Giving up on yourself can never be an option.

Dealing with failures can be particularly hard for dieters. As we discussed earlier, more than other groups dieters are subject to the what-the-hell effect when they break rank for the day, completely abandoning their efforts and better judgment. It can also be discouraging when a substantial weight-loss effort comes undone once their pre-diet habits come back to haunt them. The way to overcome these hurdles is to approach your health with the right frame of mind.

In her book *Mindset: The New Psychology of Success,* Carol Dweck describes two distinct worldviews that impact how we approach challenges: the *fixed mindset* and the *growth mindset.*[8] Someone with a fixed mindset believes that people are born with a specific set of qualities and there is little that can be done to change them. This means either you are smart or you're not, you're good at something or you're not, you have willpower or you don't, you're thin or you're fat. With these destinies sealed in stone, exerting effort to make a change is a pointless endeavor (unless it reinforces your predetermined awesomeness). In contrast, someone with the growth mindset believes that innate abilities can always be improved upon and that the key to success is concentrating efforts in the right places. As a result, people with the growth mindset have the attitude that they can improve at anything if they try hard enough and that failure is a learning experience and opportunity to grow and improve. People with the fixed mindset, on the other hand, view failure as a reflection of self-worth.

A FOODIST'S MINDSET

Foodists have a growth mindset. We believe that everyone can get healthy and lose weight. This doesn't mean that if we change our eating habits we can all look like Adriana Lima or Dwight Howard, but it does mean that we can feel and look our best and that our health destiny is in our control.

One of the most striking lessons I've learned since changing the way I approach food is that almost all the barriers we believe are keeping us from our goals are smaller and softer than we imagine. For instance, when I started buying most of my produce at the farmers market, I avoided the fruits and vegetables I didn't like as a child because I assumed my food preferences were something I was born with, and I had no interest in forcing myself to eat beets just because they were healthy. But since that time I've taught myself to not just like but *love* beets, eggplant, cucumbers, cilantro, spinach, and even brussels sprouts. All it took was understanding that my past experiences with these foods weren't representative of what I might find when I tasted them fresh and in season from the farmers market.

I now have the pleasure of enjoying instead of avoiding all these foods, making ordering at restaurants way easier and life more fun in general. Of course, I didn't just make a decision and start liking these vegetables overnight. It took effort. Brussels sprouts were by far the hardest, and I spent months trying and retrying different recipes and preparations before I was finally able to enjoy them (see recipe, p. 168). But I found the challenge fun, because I knew from my experiences with eggplant and cilantro how much I was probably missing out on by continuing to shun those little green orbs.

Those with a growth mindset also know that it's okay to not always eat perfectly healthy, which, as we've seen, is virtually impossible anyway. Instead, foodists strive to make gradual, but constant improvements in their habits that slowly mold them into fit and healthy people over time. Rather than wasting willpower on resolving battles between desires and aspirations, foodists make room for occasional indulgences, because life is too short to turn down every cupcake that crosses your path.

Never forget that eating foods you enjoy is not a bad thing—in fact, it should be your goal. And you should love all the foods you eat, healthy or otherwise. It can sometimes be hard to remember, but even those unplanned late-night pizza runs are valuable for learning about yourself and sculpting a lifestyle that works for you in the long term (maybe you need to eat more carbohydrates during the day or adopt strategies to drink less alcohol when you go out). In those moments when it feels as though you're slipping backward instead of progressing forward, think of your situation as what Homer Simpson would call a "crisitunity," after his daughter Lisa reminds him that "the Chinese use the same word for crisis as they do for opportunity." Setbacks don't define you; they are how you learn to improve. In this way not only does being a foodist eliminate your reliance on willpower; it also frees you from guilt.

The moment you stop dieting, you free up a tremendous amount of willpower that can be put to better use by focusing on building behaviors that last. The thinnest, healthiest people don't diet, because they never let their weight get out of control in the first place. Instead, they rely on dozens of small but consistent habits that, when combined, allow them to easily control their weight without much thought or effort. They understand that eating a plate of spinach doesn't make you healthy, just as eating a cookie doesn't make you unhealthy. Your health and weight are not defined by one moment in time, but are a reflection of all the things you've done to impact your body throughout your life. This way of thinking is fundamentally different from that of the chronic dieter, and it embodies the foodist's mindset.

THREE

HEALTHSTYLE

A Kinder, Gentler Way to Lose Weight and Keep It Off

"The easier it is to do, the harder it is to change."
—ENG'S PRINCIPLE

"It was when I found out I could make mistakes that
I knew I was on to something."
—ORNETTE COLEMAN, AMERICAN JAZZ MUSICIAN

In late 2008 I decided to launch Summer Tomato, a website dedicated to helping people lose weight without dieting. But when I started building the site's content, I ran into a problem. How do you talk about eating and weight loss without using the word "diet"?

In popular culture the word "diet" is synonymous with willpower and restriction, which as we've seen are the enemies of long-term success. But the word "diet" technically describes the foods that a person, animal, or community habitually eats. When we talk about a healthy diet, a canine diet, or a Western diet, this technical definition is the one we are using. Keeping the two definitions separate is nearly impossible when writing about food and weight loss. In the context of health, the word "diet" also limits the scope of our discussion to the specific foods you eat. This can be misleading, though, since the when, where, how, and why of eating (not to mention physical activity and mental well-being) are also essential factors in achieving your goals. My solution was to come up with a new word altogether.

HEALTHSTYLE

Instead of "diet," I use the word "healthstyle" to refer to the actions, dietary or otherwise, that impact your health and body weight. Your healthstyle is a reflection of your cumulative habits, from the food you eat, to how often you exercise, to where you live and the company you keep. Unlike a trendy weight-loss diet, your healthstyle is not temporary. It is neither a momentary state of being nor a vague end point, but a permanent, inescapable part of your existence. Another advantage over the word "diet" is that the term "healthstyle" acknowledges that your health is inextricably tied to your style and personality and that people can achieve good health in many different ways.

An ideal healthstyle won't look the same for everyone. Some people adore spending time in the kitchen and can craft habits around this skill. I am not one of those people, but I've found a balance of grocery shopping, making food at home, and eating out that works for me and my family. Other people hate the gym, but love swimming and spending time outdoors. No matter what your preferences, working to gradually nudge your healthstyle in a positive direction is the secret to lasting success.

Healthstyle is about the big picture, not sweating the small stuff, and having the flexibility to make changes when life throws you curve balls. The challenge is maintaining enough structure in your routines to keep you on the right path, while still giving yourself some wiggle room around the edges. What gives your healthstyle that structure is healthy habits. Because habits are consistent behaviors and not single actions, they are the only truly reliable way to make lasting improvements in your health and physique.

I'll give you step-by-step instructions on how to identify the habits that have the biggest impact on your health. We will then work to extinguish or reprogram those that are hindering your success, while continuing to develop and expand those that help. The results may not come as rapidly as they would on an arbitrary restriction diet, but they will last because they are built on a foundation of activities you enjoy, custom-tailored to your own life and needs.

YOUR BRAIN ON AUTOPILOT

Building and breaking habits will present different challenges for everyone, but one thing all habits have in common is where they begin: the brain.

Autopilot is your brain's favorite gear. Scientists estimate that up to 90 percent of our daily food choices are the result of habitual actions rather than conscious thought. This isn't because we're lazy. Decision making requires a substantial amount of mental energy and, like willpower, frequent choices quickly deplete glucose stores in our brains, a phenomenon psychologists refer to as *decision fatigue.* To streamline the decision-making process, our brains are expert at recognizing patterns and programming automatic responses, thereby saving our mental resources for novel situations. Because they work unconsciously, habits are your secret weapon for sidestepping willpower and bad decisions, allowing you to get past your weaknesses and painlessly achieve your goals.

Habits automate your actions for most (and therefore the most important) of your food choices. Automation is essential for any long-term goal that requires frequent decisions, because it takes willpower out of the equation and reduces your opportunity for failure. Do you rely on willpower and good intentions to have enough money left over at the end of each pay period to contribute to your savings? Some people try this, but most fail. It's incredibly easy to rationalize what feel like minor indulgences when it comes to things like food and money, which require dozens of small decisions each day.

Most of us learn the hard way that without establishing parameters for our behaviors it is virtually impossible to make any progress. So successful savers set up automatic deductions from their checking accounts at the beginning of every month, putting enough into savings to build a retirement fund and pay taxes at the end of the year. Similarly, building habits to automate your most frequent food decisions is more effective than restrictive dieting for achieving your long-term health and weight-loss goals—the healthstyle equivalent of your savings account. The more habits you develop that contribute to your health account automatically, the more freedom you'll have to indulge yourself every now and then without guilt, and the less willpower you need overall.

EATING FOR PLEASURE

Building healthy habits reduces the need for willpower in another way as well. For a foodist occasional treats are harmless, even welcome additions to your healthstyle. This is because focusing on long-term health eliminates the need to restrict any single food (or nutrient) and gives you a huge psychological advantage over typical diets.

Simply knowing that something is forbidden keeps it at the forefront of your mind, making it almost impossible to ignore. It's like the famous experiment by Daniel Wegner in which you are instructed to not think of a white bear. Inevitably a polar bear pops into your mind, usually within seconds or minutes—and polar bears aren't nearly as enticing as tasty food. When the forbidden action is something you know you enjoy, like eating chocolate or the amazing pizza at the place down the street, you don't stand a chance.

Most diet plans attempt to combat these breakdowns by offering phony indulgences that aren't quite as "bad" as inhaling an entire cheesecake, sad concoctions that are chemically sweetened, artificially fattened, and culinarily criminal. Nothing made with Splenda is a real treat, because it can never come close to providing the satisfaction of a real brownie made from natural butter, high-quality chocolate, and real sugar. Because your subconscious knows this, eating those fake monstrosities still requires willpower. Products like fat-free cookies and low-carb pancake mix succeed because our desperate brains try to convince our bored palates that these impostors are better than nothing in our state of deprivation. But we can only endure this sort of delusion for so long before our senses rebel and our will breaks down. Building healthy habits breaks this cycle by freeing you from the illusion that you need to eat perfectly 100 percent of the time. For chronic dieters, this idea can be hard to swallow. Though you may assume that having a license to eat what you enjoy will encourage you to binge, in practice it produces the opposite effect by reducing your need for willpower and giving you the strength to make rational, moderate indulgences on a regular basis.

With this attitude, food choices transform from a test of willpower into a question of value. Office birthdays, trips to your favorite sandwich shop, and date nights with your partner mean different things to different people. I once worked in a lab* where everyone's birthday was celebrated with a cake from one of San Francisco's premier pastry shops, Tartine Bakery. The cakes from Tartine are mind-blowing, and when I worked in the lab I actually considered birthdays excellent opportunities to bond with my fellow lab mates and indulge in some culinary bliss—it's not every day you get to eat a cake from Tartine. But I've also worked in places where office birth-

---

*This lab was aptly referred to as "The Pleasure Lab," a happy coincidence of being under the direction of principle investigator Dr. Samuel Pleasure.

days were celebrated with stale grocery-store cakes garnished with gobs of unnaturally colored, sickeningly sweet frosting. The difference was night and day. I never felt as though I was missing anything by opting out of the nasty generic cake, knowing better things were waiting for me in the future. When you know you aren't missing out and real treats are never off-limits, exercising this small amount of self-control hardly feels like a sacrifice. In fact, telling yourself that you can have any treat you like at a future time is a proven strategy to eat less and save willpower.

In their book *Willpower*, Baumeister and Tierney recommend that people who want to lose weight should "never say never." This recommendation is based on the research of Nicole Mead and Vanessa Patrick, who designed an experiment to test what would happen if they asked volunteers to resist a bowl of M&M candies that were available while they watched a short film. Some were asked to imagine they would never be able to eat them, while others were asked to skip them now, but imagine they could have as many as they wanted later. For comparison there was a control group who were allowed to eat as much as they wanted during the film. Later, the researchers asked the participants to fill out questionnaires and as a casual afterthought offered the remaining M&Ms, telling each of the unsuspecting volunteers, "You're the last subject we have today, and everyone else has gone, so these are left over. Help yourself."

Of course, the researchers were intensely interested in how each group would respond to the "Help yourself" invitation, fully expecting those who had imagined they could have the treats later to indulge to their heart's content. To their surprise, those who postponed the indulgence ended up eating significantly less than those who imagined they could never have the candies. They even ate less than those who were allowed to eat the candy at will during the film. According to Mead, "Depriving yourself of something you crave starts an internal battle that your mind will not let go of. But telling yourself you can have it later is as good as allowing yourself to have it now, because you are liberated from the internal conflict (and don't incur as many calories or feelings of psychological guilt). Postponement of a treat to some unspecified time is psychologically freeing."[1]

The tremendous implication of this research is that you can both eat less and end your cravings (i.e., feel happier about your decision) by simply telling yourself you can eat whatever you want, just not right now. When I spoke to Mead about her experiments, she said that the effect of postponing a treat reduces cravings for up to a week after the opportunity was presented. The experiment was also effective when repeated with cookies, ice cream, and potato chips, though postponing one kind of treat (e.g., chocolate) did not reduce cravings for a different kind (e.g., potato chips). The other major implication of this work is that the psychological act of depriving yourself is not effective at controlling your eating once you abandon your willpower. Indeed, those who told themselves they could never eat the M&Ms ate more when they were given the opportunity than those who allowed themselves to eat freely from the beginning. "This is consistent with previous work showing that deprivation is effortful and can backfire," said Mead. Once again we see that dieting doesn't work and that it is more effective to make value-based decisions on what and when to eat rather than outright depriving yourself.

As you can imagine, this kind of self-regulating healthstyle is far easier to deal with socially than any rigid eating plan. Strict, joyless diet rules take the fun out of life, because they lack flexibility. You shouldn't have to miss out on anything of value simply because you want to drop a few pounds or be healthy. Sure, you can spend the rest of your life eating burgers without buns if you like, but there is no need to be so extreme. Making room for these occasional indulgences not only makes socializing more fun and less awkward; it also conserves your willpower for when you really need it—that is, for establishing habits in the first place.

MAKING CHANGES: THE ELEPHANT AND THE RIDER

In their book *Switch: How to Change Things When Change Is Hard,* Dan and Chip Heath discuss the two main forces that motivate humans to act: the executive brain and the emotional brain.[2] They illustrate this with an analogy of a person riding an elephant. The rider represents the executive brain, which attempts to steer the stronger and more stubborn elephant, the emotional brain, down the right path. The rider is rational and logical, has a clearer understanding of the situation, and is responsible for planning and giving direction. But although the rider is necessary for guiding the elephant in the right direction, the logical part of the brain is powerless to make meaningful progress without the tremendous force of the emotional brain.

The elephant's temperament is very different from the rider's. It can be lazy, hedonistic, and skittish, but is also motivated by lofty ideals such as love and loyalty. The elephant is also much stronger than the rider, and if there is a conflict between the two, the elephant will usually win. When you try a diet and can't stick with it, it is not your will that fails— it is the elephant fighting back. The secret to a successful healthstyle is getting your elephant and your rider working together again.

To get the elephant working for you, it is essential to lead the elephant in a direction it wants to go. If you set goals that are too difficult or detract from (rather than add to) your quality of life, you cannot expect the elephant to play along for any meaningful amount of time. The most effective goals will satisfy the rider's desire for good health and an attractive body as well as the elephant's lust for good times and delicious food.

BUILDING HABITS

Like Rome, habits are not built in a day. Depending on the level of difficulty for the individual, a given habit can take anywhere from two weeks to eight months to develop, but on average takes about two months, or sixty-six days, to take root. Simply knowing how habits are formed makes it easier to accomplish your goals. But to fully grasp how this works, you must first have a clear understanding of what exactly a habit is.

In a nutshell, a *habit* is an automatic reaction to a specific cue or stimulus. The difference between habits and other behaviors is that the actions following the cue occur automatically rather than consciously. Because habits occur at the subconscious level, very little information is required for the action to be initiated.

Habitual behaviors can be cued by either external or internal triggers. If you have the habit of getting popcorn and a soda every time you go to the movies, the theater (more specifically the smell of buttered popcorn and the sight of the concession stand) is your cue that initiates a series of behaviors starting with getting in line and ending with munching on the buttery snack and sipping the sweet drink throughout the film. The most obvious kinds of cues are environmental, such as seeing a bowl of chips in the lunchroom or a diet-soda commercial that reminds you how nice it would be to have one right about now. But social events can also initiate automatic behavior, which is one reason smokers tend to reach for their pack when drinking coffee or alcohol. Internal cues such as emotions or moods can trigger habitual behavior as well.

Habits are *conditioned behaviors,* meaning that they develop over time with repetition and are associated with a reward or pleasurable experience, at least in the beginning. Thus successful habit building requires choosing a salient cue, deciding upon a rewarding response, and then consciously repeating this behavior until it becomes automatic. The rider—and our elusive willpower—are necessary for the first two steps, but if they are effective, the elephant will eventually take control and a habit will be born.

ENGINEERING YOUR ENVIRONMENT

Manipulating environmental cues is the easiest and often the most effective way to build better habits. The authors of *Switch* call this "tweaking your environment," or arranging your life so that it is more conducive to accomplishing your goals. In the diet space, no one has better (or more amusing) illustrations of how this works than Cornell scientist Brian Wansink. In his brilliant book *Mindless Eating: Why We Eat More Than We Think,* Wansink offers dozens of examples of how tiny, imperceptible changes in our environment can mean hundreds of extra calories every day.[3] He argues that adjustments of this kind contribute to what he calls the *mindless margin,* a 100- to 200-calorie buffer zone where our brains cannot detect the difference between more or less food. Over time calories in the mindless margin add up as weight gained or lost. Using the mindless margin to your advantage is yet another way to shrink your reliance on willpower and get control of your healthstyle.

Since some of the same environmental cues that result in overeating can be flip-flopped to cause you to eat less or make better food choices, Wansink recommends using the mindless margin to "mindlessly eat better." For example, there are dozens of ways to influence portion sizes or how much food you consume in one sitting that have nothing to do with hunger. Americans, and dieters in particular, are more inclined to use cues like an empty plate or the end of a television show to indicate that a meal is over. When smaller plates are used or 20 percent less food is served, diners will voluntarily eat less without reporting any difference in fullness or satisfaction. Most won't even notice. Using smaller plates, taller glasses, and smaller serving utensils; eating at a table instead of in front of the TV; dimming the lights; and eating more slowly can all have a significant impact on how much food you eat, and I'll explain how and when to use these strategies throughout the book.

10 Simple Ways to Eat Less Without Noticing

1. Use smaller plates

Regardless of the actual quantity of food, a full plate sends the signal that you're eating a full meal, and a partially empty plate looks like a skimpy meal.

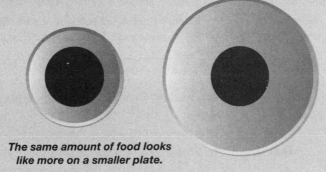

*The same amount of food looks
like more on a smaller plate.*

Using smaller plates and filling them up is a proven way to eat less without noticing.

2. Serve yourself 20 percent less

The mindless margin is about 20 percent of any given meal. In other words, you can eat 80 percent of the food you'd normally eat and probably not notice it as less, so long as no one points it out to you. You could also eat 20 percent more—not a bad idea if you're scooping vegetables. If you have those smaller plates mentioned above, serving yourself a little less should be just as satisfying.

3. Use taller glasses

Just as less food looks like more food on a smaller plate, height makes things look larger than width does, even when the volumes are the same. You can cut down on your liquid calories by choosing taller glasses rather than shorter, fatter ones.

4. Eat protein for breakfast

People love to hype eating breakfast as a miracle weight-loss cure, but only breakfasts high in protein have been proven to suppress appetite and reduce subsequent eating throughout the day. Skip the waffles and head to the omelet station instead.

5. Eat three meals a day

People often say that eating many small meals is better than eating three bigger ones throughout the day, but the data tell us otherwise. Though skipping meals can make controlling your appetite more difficult, eating more than three meals a day has not been shown to have any benefit and may even be worse for appetite control. Eat when you're supposed to and you shouldn't need any extra food.

6. Keep snacks out of sight or out of the building

Study after study has shown that people eat a lot more when food is visible rather than put away where it can't be seen, even if they know it is there. Research has also demonstrated that the harder food is to get to, even if the extra effort is just removing a lid or walking to the cabinet, the less likely you are to eat it. The extra work forces you to question the value of your action, and this gives you the opportunity to talk yourself out of a decision you may regret later.

To avoid extra snacking, keep tempting foods out of sight or, better yet, out of the house. On the flip side, keep healthy foods prominently displayed and easy to reach.

7. Chew thoroughly

Once you start paying more attention to eating speed, you may be horrified to observe that most people don't chew. If you're one of those who chew the minimum number of times before swallowing or shoveling in another forkful, chances are you're eating substantially more at every meal than your thoroughly chewing peers. Slow down, chew each bite (counting your chews can help develop the habit), and watch as you fill up faster on fewer calories.

8. Don't eat from the package

Your stomach can't count. When you can't see how much you're eating, you're more than a little likely to lose track and consume double or even triple the amount you'd eat if you took the time to serve yourself a proper portion. Use a plate, a bowl, or even a napkin. Just make sure you get a good visual of everything you're going to eat before taking your first bite.

9. Don't eat in front of the TV

For the vast majority of us, distracted eating is overeating. The end of a show or movie is another powerful cue signifying that a meal is over, so parking in front of the TV with your plate for a *Battlestar Galactica* marathon is probably not the best idea. With the invention of DVR, there's no reason you can't take thirty minutes to sit down and have a proper meal before enjoying your shows.

10. Don't pay attention to health claims

But wait, isn't healthy food supposed to be better for you? In theory, yes. But truly healthy food—vegetables, fruits, and other unprocessed foods—rarely have labels at all. Instead, foods with health claims tend to be processed junk repackaged as better-for-you alternatives.

Even worse, research from Wansink's lab has shown that people drastically underestimate the number of calories in foods with visible health claims on the packaging. People also tend to eat more food overall as a result of this miscalculation. He refers to this effect as the "health halo," and it's a recipe for packing on the pounds. For real health, stick to humble foods without labels.

Your environment can also influence what types of foods you eat. You know that box of doughnuts sitting in the middle of the table during your meeting? Closing the lid or moving the box to the table behind you will make it far less likely that you'll reach for one (or two). Keeping unhealthy foods out of sight is a proven way to limit how often you eat them. Similarly, putting fruits and vegetables on the counter or in a conspicuous place in the fridge can encourage healthier eating. Wansink's research team did an experiment in a school cafeteria where fruit sales more than doubled after they were moved to a more prominent location and displayed in colorful, inviting bowls. For a similar effect, shop at farmers markets where fresh, beautiful produce begs you to bring it home, read healthy cookbooks and food blogs with stunning food photography, and keep your kitchen and refrigerator clean and orderly.

Language is another powerful tool for making healthy foods more appealing. Would you rather eat a "healthy salad" or a bowl of "crisp baby greens tossed with a cilantro-lime vinaigrette, salmon, sweet corn, and heirloom tomato"? Most of us will choose tasty over healthy any day of the week, and being aware of the power of language cues and context is one more tool you can use to improve your healthstyle.

BREAKING HABITS

But what about cues that trigger unhealthy actions? As mentioned above, sometimes simply eliminating cues that elicit an unwanted response (like that cursed bowl of M&Ms taunting you from the corner of your desk) is sufficient to extinguish a bad habit. For this reason, many people successfully reduce their intake of unhealthy snacks by simply removing them from their house and office. If the temptations can't be moved, like the convenience store down the street that stocks your favorite flavor of ice cream, altering your behavior to reduce your exposure (try taking a different route home from work) can cut down your need for willpower and therefore the number of times you give in and bring a pint home.

That said, some studies have shown that avoidance tactics are not as effective when the bad habit is already very strong. In these cases it can help to use a kind of mental reprogramming that psychologists refer to as *counterconditioning.* Instead of trying to cut out a bad habit completely, plan to take a different action whenever you encounter the cue. For example, if you have the habit of scooping yourself a bowl of ice cream and sitting down to watch your favorite show every night after dinner, try replacing the ice cream with something healthier, like your favorite fruit. Though fruit isn't quite as indulgent as ice cream, most people enjoy it, and its subtle sweetness can satisfy your desire for an after-dinner treat.

For counterconditioning to work, it is important that you give yourself clear, specific instructions for accomplishing the correct action. For instance, in the example of replacing ice cream with fruit, you cannot expect to be successful if there is plenty of ice cream in the house but no fruit. You must therefore tell yourself that next time you go to the grocery store you will buy strawberries and forgo the ice cream (grocery shopping is one of the best times to make use of the willpower you do have—I don't recommend shopping while hungry). You could even imagine yourself cutting up the strawberries into smaller pieces so that you can eat them from a bowl with a spoon. Visualizing how you will accomplish your goals is one of the most effective ways to build new habits and is particularly powerful if you construct your plans in an *If . . . then* format: "If I want something sweet after dinner, then I will eat strawberries instead of ice cream."

Amazingly, simply identifying cues, scripts, and rewards can help you reshape your habits. In his book *The Power of Habit,* Charles Duhigg describes the Golden Rule of Habit Change.[4] Successfully swapping out a bad habit for a better one requires pairing the same cue with the same reward, but scripting a different set of actions to achieve it. In a clever short video associated with the book, Duhigg illustrates the Golden Rule of Habit Change with an anecdote about how he was able to break a daily cookie habit that caused him to put on eight pounds.

By paying more attention to and tracking his habit, he realized that the cue for his cookie craving struck at around 3:30 P.M. every day. At that time he would stand up, walk to the elevator, go up to the cafeteria, buy a chocolate chip cookie, and then eat it while socializing with colleagues. To identify the reward, he performed a series of experiments on himself. First, he tried getting up from his desk at 3:30 and taking a walk around the block. The next day he took his normal trip to the cafeteria, but bought a candy bar instead of a cookie and then took it back to his desk to eat it. On the third day he left his desk at 3:30 and went to the cafeteria, but instead of buying anything he just chatted with colleagues for ten minutes and then went back to his desk.

This way he tested whether it was the physical activity, the need for something sweet, or the socializing that he was craving at 3:30 each day. It turned out he was happiest after forgoing the cookie and chatting with friends. Thus the reward was not the sweets, but the socializing. To replace his cookie habit he now gets away from his desk every day at 3:30, talks for about ten minutes with a friend nearby, and then goes back to his desk to resume work. Since changing this habit he has lost twelve pounds.

REINFORCEMENT

New behaviors are only as effective as your elephant's willingness to follow them. As we have seen, your rider's commands (i.e., your best intentions) are insufficient as a source of long-term motivation. If the action you want to perform in response to a given cue provokes a negative or even neutral experience, don't expect your elephant to keep at it. Unfortunately, this includes subtle, or secondary, forms of negative reinforcement as well. Your elephant may initially be willing, but may become easily discouraged when actions are difficult or take too much time. For example, if you would like to develop the habit of cooking more at home, not only is it important that you enjoy the food you make; you must also be sure you don't choose recipes that require too much effort or exceed your skill level by too great a margin. When establishing new habits, start simple and be consistent until the action becomes automatic. You can always build on what you've done, but if you lose your elephant's attention, it can be difficult to get it back.

Contrary to what you might expect, explicit incentives, such as monetary rewards for good behavior, are often less effective than more subtle psychological rewards. In other words, enjoying your meal is better than putting the money you saved by cooking at home into your vacation fund. In Duhigg's cookie experiment, identifying the appropriate reward was the most important step in changing his habit. This is why I recommended strawberries instead of carrot sticks for replacing your ice-cream habit. If it is just sweetness you crave, fruit should be a sufficient replacement, because the reward is the same. To test an alternative hypothesis, you could scoop yourself some ice cream, then sit at a table without the TV on. If the ice cream is suddenly less appealing, the television may be the real reward you were craving, and sitting down to watch TV with a mug of herbal tea may be an effective, calorie-free alternative. Since repetition is the key to habit formation, positive reinforcement is an essential ingredient in building a successful healthstyle. Being able to identify salient rewards is therefore one of the most critical steps in making changes stick.

Interestingly, reinforcement is less important in affecting behavior once a habit has been formed. In one study, scientists evaluated the popcorn-eating habits of university students while at the movies.[5] They later offered them popcorn while watching music videos in either a cinema or a meeting room. Although all the students ate more popcorn in the cinema setting than in the meeting room (confirming the power of environmental cues to trigger eating habits), there was a marked difference between those who had a strong habit of eating popcorn at the movies and those who did not. Unknown to the students, half of them were served squeaky, stale popcorn, and the other half were served the fresh stuff. Those with the strong popcorn-eating habit ate the same amount of popcorn regardless of its freshness, whereas those with the weak popcorn habit ate significantly less stale popcorn than fresh popcorn. A strong habit made the students oblivious to the bad taste of old popcorn. What we can conclude from this is that once a habit is firmly established, the strength of the reward is less important.

CHOOSING HABITS

Despite what we know about cues, repetition, counterconditioning, and reinforcement, habit building is still more of an art than a science. One reason is that we are notoriously bad at identifying the environmental, social, and emotional cues that trigger our habits in the first place. Also, too frequently we forget about the elephant and attempt to instill habits based on the well-meaning but unrewarding goals of the rider. Fortunately, behavioral modification scientists have shown that being smart about which habits you choose to work on can greatly improve your chances of success.

First and foremost, always remember that motivating the elephant is your biggest obstacle. The elephant is lazy and doesn't want to do a ton of work for a small benefit. It also likes to see clear signs of progress along the way, so it knows its time is not being wasted. To avoid biting off more than your elephant can chew, start by building on things that are already working for you. Dan and Chip Heath call this looking for "bright spots," places in your life or environment where you're already making progress toward your goals. Frequently these bright spots are an excellent foundation for making significant improvements in your healthstyle. If you're a whiz in the kitchen, cooking is a great place to focus. If you're Mr. Social at the office, maybe you can steer the crew to a healthier lunch spot. Take advantage of the good weather in your city by planting a garden, making regular trips to your local farmers market, or spending more time outdoors.

I noticed that I had put on about five pounds after I finished my graduate program and started working from home. Even though I was still working out at the gym four to six days a week, my walking had decreased by two to three miles a day,* because I was no longer commuting to the lab. To solve the problem I turned to my puppy, Toaster. I was already walking him regularly, but the walks were usually short, so I could get back to work. It is easy to cut out what feel like unnecessary actions when they are not an essential part of your day—walking the dog versus getting to the office. But once I realized I needed to be less sedentary, I started taking him a little farther to the bigger dog park up the hill. In just four weeks I noticed a difference in how my clothes were fitting, and both Toaster and I had better days because of it. The extra time and effort were well worth it, and both my rider and my elephant were satisfied with the results. My bright spot was that I was already walking my dog several times a day, but your bright spots may not be so obvious. Monitoring and tracking your behavior are the most effective ways to identify bright spots in your current habits.

Another important factor in successful habit building is choosing simple, specific goals that can be accomplished with a straightforward set of actions. For example, "Eat more vegetables" is a less useful goal than "Eat green vegetables every day with lunch and dinner." These clear goals are effective because there is no wiggle room; either you accomplish your mission or you don't. When you can clearly define whether your goals are met, your progress is easier to track and you have a better understanding of what is and isn't effective. This not only helps you catch failures sooner, allowing you to adjust the course if necessary; it also gives you a sense of accomplishment as you build on your successes over time, keeping you motivated and inspired.

As I mentioned earlier, planning the specific actions you will take in response to a given cue enables you to visualize how you will succeed. In the previous example, success means making sure your lunch and din-

---

*Importantly, I would have not known this without my pedometer tracking my every move. Monitoring is hugely beneficial for healthstyle troubleshooting.

ner plates have green vegetables on them every day. For this to happen, you also need to consider where you commonly eat those meals and how those greens might get on your plate. If you eat at home, you need to go grocery shopping in order to have fresh vegetables in the house, so it helps to visualize yourself going to the store on weekends after dropping your kids off at practice. If you eat at work, you need to bring those vegetables from home. If you eat in restaurants, you need to think more carefully about how you order or consider choosing a new spot. This is why in the early stages of upgrading your healthstyle some of the most important habits to develop are regular shopping trips, preferably to the farmers market, since the elephant prefers the pleasant atmosphere and tastier food. If you are very new to healthy eating and cooking, your plan may also involve buying appropriate kitchen equipment and stocking your pantry (we will cover all of these things in later chapters).

When scripting how you will meet your goals, do your best to anticipate any obstacles that might prevent you from succeeding. For example, going to the gym on your lunch break might sound like a great way to get healthy, but if it means you don't get to eat lunch or have to eat something less satisfying, then it will be hard to sustain. Don't try to do too much at once, and start with tasks you know you can do. Tackling two or three new habits at a time is a reasonable number to start with. Taking on more than that requires too much mental energy and will sabotage your efforts.

It's not always clear which habits you should focus on when considering specific problems in your healthstyle. For instance, you may know that the lunch you eat at work every day is really unhealthy and makes it difficult for you to make progress. But if you have an office culture that is not conducive to bringing your lunch every day, it's easy to get frustrated, give up, and blame your job or your coworkers for your pizza gut, assuming nothing can be done. Usually, however, obstacles are more mental than physical. To get over these hurdles, remember to maintain the foodist's growth mindset. Focus on solutions to your problems and what you can control rather than things you can't. There are a million reasons why you can't do something to improve your life, but all that matters is the one thing you can do.

To find a solution, it can help to reexamine the true purpose of your goal. The reason for bringing your lunch to work is not to eat more home-cooked food, but to improve the quality of 30 percent of your weekday meals. Eating home-cooked food is a very effective way to accomplish this, but it is not the only way. If your coworkers order pizza every day, try ordering a side salad and eating half the pizza you normally would or recommending a different restaurant a couple of times a week. What works for someone else may not work for you, so there is no reason to limit yourself to cookie-cutter solutions.

Finally, keep an eye out for easy targets that have a large potential benefit. How attached are you to your soda habit? If you swapped it out for unsweetened tea, coffee, or sparkling water, would you be heartbroken? Small wins add up; focus on places where small adjustments create the biggest impact and build from there. If you manage to lose only one pound each week (considered very slow by typical diet standards), by the end of the year you will have lost nearly fifty pounds. I'll provide you with plenty of tips and tricks that work for me and my readers, but sometimes you'll need to be creative. And remember that if your first attempt doesn't work, you haven't failed—you just haven't succeeded yet.

FOUR

EAT FOOD

WHY YOU DON'T NEED A PH.D. TO MAKE SMART FOOD DECISIONS

"We are living in a world today where lemonade is made from artificial flavors and furniture polish is made from real lemons."
—ALFRED E. NEUMAN, MASCOT OF *MAD* MAGAZINE

"Food is an important part of a balanced diet."
—FRAN LEBOWITZ, AMERICAN AUTHOR

"Don't eat anything your great-grandmother wouldn't recognize as food."
—MICHAEL POLLAN, *IN DEFENSE OF FOOD*

If you're confused about what to eat, you're not alone. Media headlines contradict themselves every other week about which foods are healthy and which will kill you. Food companies intentionally mislead you with front-of-package health claims, and the U.S. Food and Drug Administration (FDA) lets them get away with it. And if you even casually follow the low-fat, low-carb roller coaster that fuels the latest weight-loss trends, you probably feel as helpless as a yak on a bicycle. It's a miracle we can feed ourselves at all with the kind of advice we're given.

WHY CAN'T WE ALL JUST GET ALONG?

Have you ever stopped and wondered why the health and diet messages are so confusing? It's not a fun thought experiment, so I don't blame you if you haven't. When it comes right down to it, the reason we hear so many different things is that nobody really knows what they are talking about. Or more precisely, most people only know a little bit about what they're talking about and project and extrapolate the rest to make a coherent story about what they believe. That isn't to say that everyone is giving you bad information or that there aren't smart people working on this problem. To the contrary, there is actually a lot we know about eating well and there are brilliant scientists* making huge strides in nutrition every year. The issue is that nutrition science is in its infancy relative to the complexities of plant, animal, and human biology, and until we know more there will continue to be an overabundance of hypothesizing.

Humans are omnivores, which means we are adapted to eat plants, fungi, and animals. The nutrients in the plant foods we consume depend on the genetics of the individual species, the quality of the soil they are grown in, and the weather conditions during that time. For animal foods, nutrient levels are dependent on what the animals eat throughout their lives and are also affected by their stress and hormone levels. Any toxins or environmental pollutants that the animals and plants are subjected to have the power to impact human health as well.

Nutrient levels of raw foods change depending on the amount of time between harvest and consumption (sometimes going up, sometimes going down), and your cooking method may destroy some nutrients while making others more available. Individual nutrients within

---

* Don't confuse scientists (Ph.D.s) and medical doctors (M.D.s). Because it is not part of their training, the vast majority of M.D.s don't know jack about nutrition.

a food do not work in isolation, but interact with each other to affect bioavailability (i.e., how our bodies are able to use them). Similarly, the nutrients in one food can interact with nutrients from another food if they are consumed in combination.

Your metabolism starts responding simply to the smell of food.* How quickly you eat and how much you chew also impact how your body handles it. Your own genetic makeup as well as your fitness level dictate how you respond to different levels and combinations of nutrients, and your digestive tract contains trillions† of microorganisms that affect what you can and cannot absorb. Individuals vary greatly in their sensitivity to different micro and macro nutrients, and all of us have different personal health and fitness goals.

One reason it is difficult to give nutrition advice is that there is no formula that will work for everybody in all situations. Moreover, we don't understand the details of most of these processes well enough to give reliable answers. Since we don't know far more than we do know, you should be skeptical of anyone claiming to have all the answers. Personally, I do my best to keep up on the science, but always with the understanding that we are several decades (possibly even centuries) away from even pretending to be able to prescribe an optimal diet for every individual, if such a thing even exists (it probably doesn't). Yet despite our gaps in understanding, we have seen that humans are incredibly adaptable to different diets and can thrive in a multitude of environments.[1] So part of what defines the best diet for you will be what your circumstances allow for. Within that framework you'll have to do some guesswork, starting with the best information you have and then experimenting on yourself to see what works.

---

*Amazingly, smell has been shown to significantly impact longevity in some species via the insulin-signaling pathway.

† Not exaggerating.

THE THINGS WE KNOW

The situation may sound grim, but there's no need to join a suicidal space cult just yet. Even without knowing the exact details of how the homofermentative metabolism of *Lactobacillus* in the human intestine impacts blood glucose, we still know enough about certain groups of foods to give us a decent idea of what does and does not constitute a healthy diet. It is also much easier to talk about whole foods (you know, those things we actually eat) than it is to discuss the individual nutrients that may or may not behave the way we expect them to once they've been eaten. Let's start with a few nutrition facts that virtually all scientists, nutritionists, and diet camps agree upon.

VEGETABLES ARE GOOD FOR YOU

Everyone agrees vegetables are good for you. Eating more vegetables is linked to lower body mass index (BMI) and less risk for heart disease, stroke, high blood pressure, cancer, diabetes, and pretty much every other diet-related disorder under the sun. Though we do not know the exact reasons why,* vegetables seem to protect us from a lot of the other bad things we do to ourselves. And though I've heard a few extremists argue that vegetables aren't as necessary as everyone claims,† it's a safe bet that vegetables do more good than harm.

REFINED STARCHES AND SUGARS ARE BAD FOR YOU

The nutrition community is one of the most disagreeable bunches in all of science. To hear the diet fundamentalists argue, you might think we

---

* There's been plenty of speculation that it's the vitamins, minerals, antioxidants, or other nutrients in vegetables that should be credited, but research has consistently shown that the benefits of vegetables tend to be eliminated when individual molecules are separated out from the whole food.

† Inuit tribe members eat very few vegetables and seem to be healthy.

were on the brink of a holy war. But across the board, from vegans like Dr. Colin Campbell to carnivores like Dr. Robert Atkins, not one of them considers refined carbohydrates to be nutritionally neutral—they all consider them dangerous. Take it to heart, because we may never see this kind of civility again.

Because they are processed, refined carbohydrates are not technically whole foods, but most of us recognize them a class of foods that includes breads, cakes, chips, sweeteners, and sodas. Their hallmark ingredients are refined flour and sugar, and it's appropriate to call this stuff junk food. You'll see that you can still save some space for them in your healthstyle, but under no circumstances should you forget that these are not health foods.

THE SUPERFOOD ILLUSION (AKA THE FINE PRINT)

Before we move on to the more controversial foods, I want to pause and reflect on what we've covered, lest we become too dogmatic and overconfident about what we actually know. I've said it's undeniable that vegetables are healthy, but that doesn't mean you should start eating celery like a health-crazed lunatic. Remember that the details of why these foods are good for us are still relatively unknown, so it's important not to fall into the "superfood illusion" and gorge yourself on a handful of select foods just because of some wonder nutrient they are supposed to possess.

I always cringe when I hear a scientist use the word "superfood," because I know it will inevitably be parroted by the media or, worse, a food company trying to sell us some bogus product. "Superfood" is a marketing term typically used to mean a plant (e.g., blueberries) or animal (e.g., salmon) that contains high levels of a particular nutrient (antioxidants! omega-3s!) that can supposedly help with a certain health issue. When something gets labeled as a superfood, most of us automatically assume it is extra super-duper healthy and we should go out of our way to eat more of it. Not that we will (according to decades of research, few people can even manage five fruits and vegetables a day), but maybe we'll try to try and eat more.

To their credit, the superfood lists I've seen usually contain legit health foods. They tend to be fruits, vegetables, fish, and other natural ingredients. Thankfully, I haven't seen any reports that bottled vitamin water is a superfood and actually good for you. But it is naive to believe there is some list of magical foods that will save you from certain death. Obviously nutrients are important (and vitamins are essential), but large doses of them from either food or supplements are almost never associated with benefits beyond what you can expect from having an overall healthy diet. This is because the way our body deals with micronutrients is not linear (i.e., more does not mean better). Instead, there is typically an ideal dose range for a given nutrient; amounts below or above this range are both bad, but any reasonable quantity in between is pretty darn good. Think of Goldilocks finding the perfect porridge temperature and bed softness. In normal ranges your nutrient levels will be just right, freeing you to go about snooping in the homes of bears (or whatever).

Though it is hard to overdose on whole foods, it is possible. In 2010, the *New England Journal of Medicine* reported that an eighty-eight-year-old woman fell into a coma after eating 2 to 3 pounds of raw bok choy each day for several months.[2] She had been attempting to control her diabetes, but instead induced a state of severe hypothyroidism. Though bok choy is typically a very healthy vegetable, when eaten raw and in large quantities some of the compounds in it break down into chemicals that inhibit the thyroid. The lesson here is that bingeing on random foods (even if you convince yourself they're healthy) isn't a good idea. But more important, eating a lot of one kind of food almost certainly won't give you any health advantage. If you're eating one thing, that means you aren't eating something else, and in Western cultures what we're really lacking is nutrient diversity.

The Top 10 Most Overrated Health Foods

Like it or not, we tend to believe whatever we are exposed to in the media and in advertisements. In nutrition this usually means that as a society we all follow the same diet fads, glorifying some foods over others in the quest for better health. (It's okay. I love salmon and coconut water as much as you do.)

The problem is, though, that more often than not the news or the health claims made by food manufacturers vastly overstate any potential health benefits, because doing so makes a more compelling story and sells more products. Our own confirmation biases tend to make us believe what we're told, we confidently share our insights with our friends, and suddenly our grocery stores are filled with health foods that really aren't all they are cracked up to be. Here are my ten picks for the most overrated health foods.

1. Yogurt

There is nothing innately wrong with yogurt, the natural product. But the real stuff is not nearly as easy to find as the hypersweetened dessert versions filling supermarket shelves. Though yogurt can contain beneficial probiotics, friendly bacteria are also present in other fermented foods like sauerkraut, kimchi, and miso. And if you are worried about acne, dairy is probably not your best choice. Oh, and the overratedness is doubly true of frozen yogurt.

If you'd rather keep yogurt as your breakfast staple (something I often use myself), go for plain yogurt, preferably full fat. Don't fall for the vanilla trap; it is not plain and has even more sugar than most fruit versions.

2. Soy

Soy is another one of those foods that can be perfectly healthy, but can also be processed into oblivion, making it an unhealthy product. Hydrogenated soy oil is among the most common sources of trans fat. Processed products are often touted as healthy just because they contain soy, but soy is not exactly the health panacea it is often made out to be. For a healthier version, stick to fermented soy products like miso, natto, or tempeh.

3. Egg Whites

It baffles me that Americans continue to vilify the most nutritious part of the egg while glorifying the less impressive half. Sure, egg whites are a good source of protein on their own, but you're probably not lacking protein and would likely benefit from the rich nutrients of the entire egg.

4. Margarine

Why we need artificial processed oils when there are so many naturally healthy sources of fat is beyond me—that is, assuming you can even find margarines that do not contain hydrogenated oils (trans fats). If you really want more stanols and sterols in your diet, try eating more nuts, avocados, and vegetables. If you want to add buttery flavor, just use real butter (preferably from grass-fed cows).

5. Bananas

I have a bit of a reputation for picking on bananas, but I really don't think they're all bad, and they definitely taste yummy. My biggest problems with them are that they are produced industrially and are one of the most calorie-dense fruits you can buy. When is the last time you saw a banana at the farmers market anyway?

Bad for you? Not really.

Overrated? Definitely.

6. Fake Meat

Next time you get a chance, check out the ingredients in your favorite meat substitute. It usually contains a lot of gluten, some processed soy, canola oil, cornstarch, and a few bizarre ingredients like "natural vegetarian flavors" (mmm . . . vegetarians). Call me crazy, but real meat sounds a lot more appealing.

7. Protein Bars

Remember back in the day when protein bars tasted like crap? Well, they would all still taste that way if manufacturers didn't fill them with sugar or sugar substitutes. Look at the ingredients. The vast majority of protein bars contain the same processed junk that's in everything else, just with a few more vitamins, some added soy protein, and possibly some added fiber. Adding nutrients to junk food does not a health food make.

8. Whole-Grain Flour

Ah, whole grains, how controversial be thy name. Though I'm not as antigrain as some folks, I don't pretend that highly processed "whole-wheat flour" is actually good for me. Grains that don't look like grains are not your friends.

9. Low-Fat Salad Dressing

Fat is good for you. Yes, fat contains more calories than protein or carbohydrates, but it also enables you to absorb more vitamins from the foods you eat and makes your meals more satisfying. Fat-free dressings do not make you healthier; they make your salad less nourishing.

10. Fruit Juice

Juicing fruit concentrates the sugar while stripping out the filling fiber. When you remember that one 450-ml (15-ounce) bottle of orange juice is equivalent to six whole oranges, you can start to see the problem. Green juices are fine; just be careful with fruit juices.

The vast majority of our diets are made up of the same handful of foods that we eat over and over again. Even people who make sincere efforts to eat healthy have rather limited diets. Broccoli, carrots, and zucchini are great and all, but it pays to be a little more creative. Throwing blueberries in there every now and then can only add so much. There are hundreds, maybe thousands of important nutrients (vitamins, antioxidants, phytochemicals, etc.) that our bodies need for optimal performance, and as we discussed earlier we probably don't know what all of them are, let alone what functions they serve. Every natural food contributes its own unique blend of nutrients, so if you want to get the most from your diet, you're much better off focusing on dietary diversity rather than loading up on the top ten foods some magazine says you should eat more of.

All that said, it does make me happy when lowly, forgotten vegetables like beets and lima beans get featured in the *New York Times*. Vegetables need all the press they can get, and it's true that most people don't eat enough vegetables, period. Any article that encourages you to try a new kind of food is a good thing. But keep in mind that if you see a food labeled "super," you should take it with a grain of salt, because when it comes down to it all natural foods are superfoods. The ones that make the news just happen to be those that some scientist or reporter decided to shine the spotlight on for the time being.

SEAFOOD IS GOOD FOR YOU (USUALLY)

Seafood marks the beginning of the healthy-eating gray area. If we had pristine rivers, lakes, and oceans, there wouldn't be much of an issue. Where the science stands today, the evidence is pretty convincing that fish and seafood, when unadulterated, are uniquely healthy. The problem arises when we consider the environmental toxins that pollute our waterways and contaminate our food as well as the ecological issues caused by overfishing. I'll address these issues separately in the following pages.

Though I prefer not to focus on individual nutrients, it is clear that seafood is rich in at least two essential omega-3 fatty acids, docosahexaenoic acid (DHA) and eicosapentaenoic acid (EPA), which are virtually

Fishing for Answers:
How to Choose Fish and Seafood

I don't think there is anything more complicated in the food world than fish and seafood. There are so many life-or-death issues, it's enough to make you want to cover your eyes, plug your ears, and live out the rest of your life in a cave on Mars. But this isn't really one of those issues we can ignore. Beyond the obvious health benefits of seafood, we must consider the consequences of environmental contaminants that accumulate in fish as well as the tragic reality of overfishing and the damage the fishing industry is doing to the environment.

Mercury

Mercury is released into the environment by chlorine plants and coal-fired power plants. Once released from a power plant, mercury settles in nearby aquatic environments, and bacteria there convert it into methylmercury. Residing at the base of the food chain, these bacteria are consumed by plankton, which are then eaten by smaller fish, which are in turn eaten by larger fish. Methylmercury has a seventy-two-day half-life, so it accumulates in animals highest on the food chain. The larger the fish, the more the methylmercury contamination. Predatory fish such as tuna, shark, swordfish, tilefish, and king mackerel have high methylmercury levels. As predatory consumers of large fish, humans are also subject to methylmercury accumulation.

The FDA warns against mercury exposure, particularly for women who are pregnant, may become pregnant, or are nursing, and children under the age of six. Methylmercury is a known neurotoxin that is able to cross the blood–brain barrier into the central nervous system and placenta. It can be dangerous for anyone exposed to high concentrations, but is particularly dangerous to children whose nervous systems are still developing. The FDA recommends that fish with high mercury content be consumed no more than once a month for normal adults and completely avoided by children and pregnant women.

For most fish consumers, tuna is the biggest concern. Bluefin, bigeye, and albacore (white) tuna contain the highest methylmercury levels. Albacore is sometimes canned, but the most common canned tuna in the United States are yellowfin and skipjack tuna. Skipjack tuna, being a much smaller fish, is relatively low in methylmercury compared to other options. It is usually labeled "chunk light tuna," but you need to read the label carefully to see that it is not yellowfin or albacore.

PCBs

Farmed fish tend to be lower in mercury concentrations, but much higher in polychlorinated biphenyls (PCBs). PCBs are chemical contaminants known to cause problems with cognition, reproduction, development, and liver function and can promote endocrine disruption. They are also thought to be carcinogenic. Though their industrial use was banned back in the 1970s, PCB contamination is widespread in American waterways and throughout the world. PCBs pose a problem because virtually all fish have some contamination, but farmed fish, particularly those fed fish meal and fish oils, tend to have more. Farmed fish are also usually less nutritious due to their limited diets. Did you know that all farmed salmon is dyed pink, because naturally it appears gray and unappetizing? Eeeew.

Basic Guidelines

For health, the basic guidelines I recommend include:

- Eat fish two or three times a week.
- Avoid large fish that accumulate mercury like tuna, shark, and swordfish.
- Avoid farmed fish that contain PCBs.
- Seek smaller fatty fish such as salmon, mackerel, and sardines.
- Avoid freshwater fish caught by friends. Almost all lakes and rivers are contaminated with high mercury levels.

Seafood Watch List

In matters of sustainability my go-to source is the Monterey Bay Aquarium's Seafood Watch List.[3] I don't know as much about the environment as I do about health, but in general I follow the guidelines below to help myself sleep at night.

BUY FROM TRUSTED SOURCES. Since I personally cannot keep up on all the fish sustainability issues, I am sure to shop at places that do. Most small, high-end seafood vendors do a good job of at least telling you where their fish comes from and will often include sustainability labels.

SHOP AT WHOLE FOODS. Though Whole Foods isn't perfect, it does a great job of labeling the origin of its animal products. This is leaps and bounds over what most grocery stores do.

EAT WILD ALASKAN SALMON. Alaskan fishing regulations are designed to promote sustainability, and their methods have been incredibly effective. Alaskan salmon is also nutritionally superior to Atlantic or farmed salmon.

EAT SARDINES. These little guys are sustainable, healthy, and delicious. I prefer fresh sardines, but I also enjoy the boneless, skinless sardines from cans. Pair with dry-as-a-bone white wine. Yum, yum.

NEVER, EVER EAT BLUEFIN TUNA. These magnificent animals are on the verge of extinction. Don't do it!

EAT FISH AT RESPONSIBLE RESTAURANTS. These days many high-end restaurants proudly label the origin of their fish on the menu. This is not always true, however, especially in Japanese restaurants.

NEVER SHOP AT CHEAP ASIAN FISH MARKETS. Cheap fish equals bad news. Sorry. I know a lot of people rely on these, but personally I do not trust them. Many of the fish sold at these stores are shipped in from China (if the store clerks deny it, they are likely lying to you). China is notorious for intentionally mislabeling its food products. Don't assume the fish from there is either safe or sustainable, regardless of what the label says.

AVOID TUNA. Do you still order maguro (tuna) at sushi restaurants? How boring and unethical. Try getting something that you've never heard of that may be less likely to be overfished. And don't be afraid to ask where it came from.

ASK THE MONTEREY BAY AQUARIUM. When in doubt, visit its Super Green List[4] for the best seafood choices at the moment.

impossible to get from other sources.* These are essential fatty acids, meaning that, like any other vitamin, you should consider them necessary for your body to function properly. Fish oils protect against heart disease and help preserve cognitive function during aging. They also help fight depression and rheumatoid arthritis and are essential for proper brain development in children. These fatty acids also have anti-inflammatory properties and have been linked with healthier digestion. With two or three servings of oily fish per week[†] all of these benefits could be yours.

WHOLE GRAINS, MEAT, AND DAIRY ARE *REALLY* CONTROVERSIAL (BUT PROBABLY FINE)

Now for the fun stuff. Want to start a fight? Walk into a paleo conference (or online forum) and tell them red meat will kill you by causing heart disease and cancer and that whole grains are healthy, especially for the heart. If you can escape without a bunch of barefoot dudes chucking you across the parking lot, you'll probably at least have a few hundred scientific articles disproving everything you were ever told hurled at you in scorn. Want to start another fight? Go to a vegan conference and tell them the exact opposite—that meat is healthy and whole grains are dangerous—and you'll get the same response, except the pile of articles flying toward your face will seem to support their argument instead.[††]

---

*Vegetarian sources of omega-3 fatty acids contain ALA (alpha-linolenic acid), but not DHA or EPA. Though technically our bodies can convert ALA to DHA and EPA, the transformation occurs so inefficiently that these cannot be considered sufficient sources of these essential molecules. ALA is healthy in its own right, but it is not a substitute for fish oil.

[†] Or a daily (1,000 mg) DHA/EPA supplement, if there's a reason you cannot eat fish.

[††] If you really want to cause some trouble, hack their websites and make it appear as if their conferences are at the same place at the same time. Don't forget your camera.

So who is right? Obviously the science isn't as clear-cut as any dogmatist would like you to believe, or the debate wouldn't be so heated. I'll start by pointing out the slightly uncomfortable fact that the majority on both sides of the fence appear to be healthy people. Sure, there are exceptions,* but for the most part these are all people who care deeply about health and what they put into their bodies. Most of them eat real food and as populations eat far more vegetables than your average Joe. Similarly, both groups eat closer to the way I eat than your typical American. From the outside, demonizing either doesn't seem like a particularly wise strategy. And I would never suggest that people change what works for them to meet some theoretical health ideal.

EATING ANIMALS

Meat is undoubtedly controversial. Beyond the ethical questions regarding using animals for food, for decades scientists and government agencies have told us that meat and its coconspirator, saturated fat, are responsible for heart disease (the number one killer in Western civilization) and recommended everyone cut way back on consumption.

After over half a century of additional research, it turns out this condemnation may have been a bit premature. In 2010, a panel of the world's leading experts on heart disease met at a conference in Copenhagen to reach a consensus on the state of the research regarding saturated fat and heart disease. The report was published in 2011 in the *American Journal of Clinical Nutrition*.[5] Contrary to what a rational person may have expected, given the recommendations over the past several decades, reducing how much saturated fat you eat is not a reliable way to reduce heart risk.

---

* To be honest I've seen more unhealthy vegans and vegetarians, but I wouldn't be surprised if this turned out to be a reflection of their larger numbers, since the paleo trend is relatively new.

This is because what you replace the fat with is important. Replacing saturated fat with carbohydrates provides no benefit, and if those carbohydrates are refined, they are actually more harmful than the animal fat. Similarly, there is not enough evidence that replacing saturated fat with monounsaturated fat (the kind in olive oil) reduces heart-disease risk. Heart protection only occurs when saturated fats are replaced with polyunsaturated fats, those lovely omega-3 fatty acids that are found in fish and some plants.* Processed oils, like those nasty trans fats we hear so much about (which can be either mono- or poly-unsaturated), are also more dangerous than saturated fats. Likewise, processed meats (think pink slime) are worse for the heart than natural meats that contain saturated fat.

Still, this does not let meat off the hook completely. This study only addressed heart disease, but cancer and other diseases may still be a concern. There is also the issue of sourcing. For instance, industrial meat production relies heavily on hormones and antibiotics to allow animals to grow bigger and faster than they ever would in nature. They are also housed in unsanitary conditions and fed grains rather than their natural diet of grass, both of which deplete the nutrient quality (not to mention flavor) of farm animals. Moreover, environmental toxins tend to accumulate in the fat of animals, so those subjected to industrial conditions may be concentrated sources of chemicals that may increase cancer and other health risks for people who eat them. We don't yet have the answers to all these questions, but I would not feel comfortable stating that you can eat unlimited amounts of meat from any source and expect it to come without consequences.

That said, meat is one of the most nutritious foods available to humans. It's rich in vitamin B_{12}, an essential nutrient not available in sufficient quantities in plant foods alone. Vegetarians must take a sup-

---

* Remember, DHA and EPA are not the only polyunsaturated fats.

plement to receive sufficient B_{12}. Meat is also an excellent source of vitamin B_6, niacin, iron, selenium, zinc, and other essential vitamins and minerals. You don't have to like it, but meat does pack a nutritional punch that's hard to beat. If you are careful about quality and keep your portions in an acceptable range,* it is reasonable to include meat as a regular part of your healthstyle. I've found that I lose weight fastest if I include some meat, but not very much. You will have to experiment to figure out the best amount for yourself.

WHOLE GRAINS

In many ways whole grains are just as controversial as meat. Entire books have been written (albeit not very convincingly) about how wheat and gluten are the cause of all the problems in Western civilization. Meanwhile, nutritionists and medical establishments are still telling us whole grains are an essential part of a healthy diet. What's the story?

One of the problems is that the science is difficult to interpret. It's easy to find studies showing that people who eat more "whole grains" (I'll explain the quotation marks shortly) are healthier in every way than people eating more refined grains. That's undeniable, and it's one of the reasons everyone agrees processed carbohydrates are bad for you. However, this fact does not prove that eating "whole grains" is better than not eating "whole grains" in the context of a healthier diet based on diverse vegetables, wild fish, and pastured meats. Another problem is that the definition of "whole grains" has been watered down to a point where it is virtually meaningless. Thanks to the FDA, the current definition of a "whole grain" is friendly to food companies, but not to consumers. The FDA requirements a manufacturer must meet to use

---

*I recommend no more than 3 to 6 ounces per serving for most people (about the size of a deck of cards), because those steak calories add up fast.

The Top 10 Most Underrated Health Foods

We already know that food manufacturers and the media tend to exaggerate the benefits of popular health foods, but what about all the wonderfully healthy foods they ignore? It's time to shine the spotlight on ten of my favorite healthy foods that never get the attention they deserve.

1. Oysters

Per calorie, oysters are one of the most nutritious foods on the planet and are particularly high in essential omega-3 fatty acids and vitamin D, which is notoriously tough to get from food. Also, because oysters lack a central nervous system and 95 percent of the world's supply is sustainably farmed, some vegetarian thought leaders have argued that oysters can be included in the diet as an ethical source of natural vitamin B_{12} (present in significant quantities only in animal foods).

2. Sauerkraut and Kimchi

I'm the first to admit that fermented foods can be a little pungent, but that doesn't preclude them from tasting delicious and being one of the healthiest things you can eat. Traditionally, fermentation has been used to preserve foods, but it also serves to increase nutritional value and add friendly bacteria to the gut. These healthy microbes help with digestion and nutrient absorption, and without them our gut health deteriorates substantially, setting the stage for many chronic diseases.

3. Dark and Organ Meats

People often demonize meats, especially the darker varieties, for their fat content and overlook how nutritious they are. Of course, they are relatively higher in calories as well, which is why you don't need to eat very much at a sitting. But fear of saturated fat shouldn't deter you from enjoying the occasional piece of fatty meat every now and then. Organ meats in particular, like liver and kidney, are rich sources of essential nutrients, and they can be delicious when prepared properly.

4. Seaweed

Okinawa is a small island in southern Japan that is home to some of the longest-lived people on earth. Sea vegetables are a staple of the traditional Okinawan diet and are thought to be responsible for many aspects of Okinawans' health. Seaweed is also a good source of iodine for people who prefer to use high-end sea salts or kosher salt for cooking, which lack sufficient iodine. I make an effort to eat seaweed often and try as many different kinds as I can get my hands on.

5. Egg Yolks

I might be beating a dead horse with this one, but until I stop seeing friends and family throwing out perfectly good egg yolks, I'm just going to keep drilling home this point. Egg consumption is not associated with heart disease. Dietary cholesterol has a negligible impact on blood cholesterol, and for some people whole eggs even improve blood lipids. Also, you're throwing away so much tasty goodness. Keep in mind that if you buy fresh, pastured eggs (hens frolicking in grass eating bugs—find them at your local farmers market or health food store), nutrient values will be significantly higher than in conventional eggs.

6. Beans and Lentils

My favorite thing about Tim Ferriss's *The 4-Hour Body* is that it made beans and lentils cool to eat.[6] I've been telling readers this for years, and finally people are listening, but there are still a lot of folks out there who don't appreciate how wonderful they really are.

For myself and many others, weight loss is much easier when we include beans and lentils rather than eliminating carbohydrates completely. Plus they fill you with energy without the bloating and other negative effects that can sometimes come from grains. They're also a great source of iron, folate, and other essential nutrients.

7. Root Vegetables

Root vegetables are right up there with the green leafies in my book. In fact, many of them are from the same cruciferous family. I never come home from shopping without at least one bunch of radishes, salad turnips, or carrots. I also have a lot of love for beets, sunchokes, and even potatoes. Vegetables don't need to be green to be good for you.

8. Coffee

Many people view their morning brew as a vice, but in reality coffee is a healthy beverage. Coffee is one of the best sources of polyphenols and antioxidants in many people's diets and has been proven to protect against liver disease, type 2 diabetes, and a host of other diseases. The biggest problem most people have with coffee is confusing the brew itself with the creamy, sugary drinks that are closer to milkshakes than health elixirs. The only real risk of too much coffee is that it can upset your sleep.

9. Hard Cheese

Yes, I just called cheese healthy. But of course I'm not talking about the processed American "cheese" that may or may not contain milk. Sadly, I'm not even talking about burrata. Hard cheeses that have been aged (think parmesan and asiago) are the most significant dietary source of vitamin K_2, a nutrient that has been shown to protect against heart disease and cancer. Like meat, cheese has a lot of calories, so you still have to be careful about how much you eat. But it's important to understand that cheese is not just empty calories, and in reasonable amounts it can actually be good for you.

10. Mushrooms

Americans tend to view mushrooms as a neutral food, but they have been used in Chinese medicine for thousands of years. Though there really isn't enough evidence to make conclusive statements about the health benefits of all mushrooms, many compounds have been identified in mushrooms that show potential for boosting immunity and possibly protecting against cancer. Mushrooms are also an unappreciated source of vitamins and minerals and shouldn't be ignored as low-calorie sponges that only go on pizza.

the term "whole grain" on its label (along with the respective health claims based on the half-truth science mentioned above) are as follows:

> Cereal grains that consist of the intact, ground, cracked or flaked caryopsis, whose principal anatomical components—the starchy endosperm, germ, and bran—*are present in the same relative proportions as they exist in the intact caryopsis*—should be considered whole grain food. (emphasis mine)

Get it? To be considered "whole," grains do not have to be intact. Thus food manufacturers create products using this loose definition to their advantage, processing grains as normal and then adding back the required ratios of grain parts (germ and bran) to meet the standard. This is how some kids' sugary cereals get spiffy health labels claiming they lower heart disease, when any unbiased nutrition scientist would agree that, with 41 percent sugar by weight, they almost certainly *contribute* to heart disease. In contrast, research has shown that when the structure of a grain is maintained there is a substantial improvement in carbohydrate metabolism.[7]

Some have made the argument that grains should be avoided completely due to the presence of "antinutrients" such as phytic acid and lectins (and yes, these people feel the same way about beans and nuts). Phytic acid (phytate) can bind up certain minerals and prevent their absorption in the body. Zinc and iron are the most problematic, and indeed phytic acid intake is sometimes associated with zinc and iron deficiencies in populations on very limited diets. However, both zinc and iron are abundant in animal products (shellfish like oysters are particularly rich in zinc), so most carnivorous Westerners are not in any danger of being deficient in these minerals. Lectins work differently, disrupting metabolism by interacting with the cells lining the gut. Though very high levels of lectins can be problematic, lesser doses do not appear to cause problems for well-nourished humans. Furthermore, anticancer properties have been attributed to both phytic acid and lectins.* If you are worried about phytic acid and lectins, sprouting, fermenting, and cooking seeds, beans, and grains can drastically reduce the concentration of antinutrients, virtually eliminating any danger.

My personal experience with grains is that, as long as the ones I choose still look like a grain (think rice, oats, farro, barley, etc.), I can eat a small serving (about a half cup) up to once or twice a day while continuing to lose weight and feel good. In fact, I find that I am happier when I include some starch in my diet (I prefer beans or lentils, but grains also suffice), since it gives me more energy and I feel far more satisfied with less food compared to when I eat vegetables and meat exclusively. Of course, what works for me will not necessarily work for everyone, and I've spoken with people who do better with less starchy foods and some who do better with more. For refined grains like breads and noodles, I've found that I can get away with one or two small servings a week and maintain my weight. However, I lose weight faster without them, and if I'm not careful with my portion sizes, bread can make me very lethargic. But I do love me some pizza every now and again. If you find yourself craving breads and sweets, intact grains or beans are a great way to kill those urges without wreaking havoc on your metabolism.

SAY CHEESE

Milk, cheese, and other dairy products are a third category of foods that get people's blood boiling. The U.S. Dairy Council has convinced all of us that milk does a body good and that we're all dying of calcium

---

* Several examples in human biology show that something that appears to be dangerous may also come with some benefits. For instance, smoking cigarettes is proven to protect against Parkinson's disease, and sickle-cell anemia protects against malaria. Once again I'll warn against overinterpreting a single scientific finding.

deficiency. Unfortunately, their marketing tactics are far stronger than the science backing their claims.

Let's start with calcium. Conventional wisdom tells us that calcium is important for strong teeth and bones, and we've been taught (falsely) that dairy is pretty much the only place to get it. Although calcium is indeed necessary, there is no evidence that eating more dairy is a reliable way to prevent bone loss.[8] In fact, osteoporosis is more common in Western countries than in Asia, Africa, or South America, where dairy is far less common (and lactose intolerance is far more common). Dairy also significantly raises men's risk of prostate cancer.[9] Calcium supplementation alone is actually associated with increased fracture risk[10] (so much for that theory) as well as heart disease. Vitamin D in combination with calcium, on the other hand, does reduce fractures.[11] Eating plenty of fruits, vegetables, fish, meat, and legumes (all excellent sources of calcium and other nutrients) are more important for bone health than dairy. On a positive note, calcium does seem to reduce the risk for colorectal cancer,[12] and claims that it promotes breast cancer have not been substantiated.

Of course, no discussion of dairy is complete without also mentioning saturated fat. Health-conscious people are often terrified by cheese and butter, because they're worried about all the saturated fat and cholesterol. Though we've already discussed how saturated fat is not reliably linked to cardiovascular disease (for the record, neither is dietary cholesterol), studies that have specifically looked at dairy have also not identified a positive association.[13] To the contrary, a few studies have shown that cheese (particularly hard cheeses) may actually be beneficial in fighting heart disease. Cheese is the primary source of vitamin K_2 (also called menaquinone, or MK-8) in the human diet.[14] Studies have repeatedly shown that individuals who consume the most menaquinone have a decreased risk of cardiovascular disease.[15] Interestingly, vitamin K_2 has also been associated with decreased risk of cancer[16] and metabolic syndrome.[17] Although there clearly needs to be

Sliced Bread Was Never a Great Invention

Food marketers have been at it for nearly a century. They're saving us time, making it ever easier for us to consume their products, and all they ask in return is to charge us a little extra for the "convenience." Aren't they sweet?

When pressed, most of us will acknowledge that the top priority of food marketers is not to make our lives easier or our food tastier, but to get us to eat (and spend) more. What's truly remarkable is that, despite knowing this, we still parrot and defend their ideas as ardently as if we'd thought of them ourselves.

Do you really believe Krispy Kreme makes the best doughnuts, Ben & Jerry's makes the best ice cream, or life is impossibly difficult without presliced bread? My guess is you probably do, or at least did at some point. But the reality is that none of these things are true, and that we think they are is just a sign of brilliant marketing.

Food isn't like other products. There are people who buy every single gadget that Apple creates, and if Apple started making twice as many products per year those people would still buy them all. But humans can only eat so much food, which makes it difficult for food companies to expand their market and be competitive.

Enter "added value."

Sliced bread, instant oatmeal, and single-serving Go-gurt are all examples of foods designed to be easier to eat. And companies correctly assume that we are happy to pay more for the free time these conveniences allot us. But does this freedom really make our lives better?

I would never argue that time doesn't have value. Though I think there is a strong case for slowing down and taking time to eat mindfully, I certainly see the appeal of fast and portable food. Having built, launched, and promoted my own website while simultaneously finishing my Ph.D., I certainly know what it means to be busy. But convenience is not the only thing you get when marketers sell you on their products. You also eat more, and you eat worse.

Because sliced bread is easier to eat, people tend to eat more of it, along with whatever they choose to put on top. Additionally, since real bread quickly becomes stale when cut into smaller pieces, food companies have had to find new (non-ecofriendly) packaging and add preservatives, dough conditioners, and other chemicals to keep breads soft. The ingredient list on a loaf of Wonder Bread is truly remarkable:

> Wheat Flour, Water, High Fructose Corn Syrup or Sugar, Yeast, Contains 2% or Less of: Ferrous Sulfate (Iron), B Vitamins (Niacin, Thiamine Mononitrate (B-1), Riboflavin (B-2), Folic Acid), Barley Malt, Soybean Oil, Salt, Calcium Carbonate (Ingredient in Excess of Amount Present in Regular Enriched White Bread), Wheat Gluten, Dough Conditioners (Sodium Stearoyl Lactylate, Mono and Diglycerides, Calcium Dioxide, Datem and/or Azodicarbonamide), Vitamin D-3, Calcium Sulfate, Vinegar, Yeast Nutrients (Monocalcium Phosphate, Dicalcium Phosphate, Ammonium Sulfate, Ammonium Phosphate and/or Ammonium Chloride), Cornstarch, Wheat Starch, Soy Flour, Whey, Calcium Propionate (to Retain Freshness), Soy Lecithin.

In contrast, the bread I buy at Acme, my local bakery, is made of flour, water, yeast, and salt. Special loaves may contain olives or herbs, but you get the general idea. I have to cut it myself, and it doesn't last long if I leave it on the counter (it freezes absolutely beautifully), but the bread at Acme is also some of the best-tasting bread I've had in my life. Are you shocked that my Acme loaf costs around $2, while Wonder Bread costs close to $4?

I don't eat much bread, because it is not particularly healthy. But I enjoy burgers, pizza, sandwiches, naan, and other traditional foods way too much to cut it out completely. Reasonable quantities of bread can easily be incorporated into a healthy diet, particularly if you exercise regularly. But bread is not health food, and eating as little as you're comfortable with is generally a good idea.

We do not need unhealthy foods to be more convenient or less expensive. And if you're going to put health aside and eat them anyway, they should also taste absolutely amazing, not just good or even pretty good. Does presliced bread really make the cut? I don't think so.

Sliced bread was never a great invention—it was great marketing. "The greatest thing since sliced bread" was derived from an ad campaign claiming its invention was "the greatest forward step in the baking industry since bread was wrapped." The phrase may be perfect for describing brilliant marketing ("The greatest added-value campaign since sliced bread"), but do we really need to continue propagating the message that low-quality convenience food is the best invention of the past one hundred years?

If we want a true benchmark for greatness, maybe we should change it to "The greatest thing since the Internet."

more research done on this topic, it seems that the theory that cheese promotes heart disease has been thoroughly debunked.*

WHAT TO AVOID

I don't like to demonize any food, but I understand that it can be helpful to know exactly which foods are problematic. Keep in mind this doesn't mean you can never eat these, just that they are not ideal for optimal health and weight loss. The following are the first things you should consider cutting back on if you're having trouble meeting your healthstyle goals.

Sugar is public enemy number one when it comes to weight loss, health, and longevity. Where there is sugar there is obesity, diabetes, heart disease, tooth decay, and cancer. Records have shown that isolated societies that have not been exposed to large quantities of sugar and flour tend to be free from these ailments, despite the fact that the people live to impressive ages. Moreover, these "diseases of civilization" were virtually nonexistent before the widespread availability of refined sugar beginning in the eighteenth century.

---

*Please do not confuse real cheese that has been fermented with the overly processed American "cheese" that may or may not actually contain milk (read the label). The fermenting process is what creates the health benefits.

One of the biggest problems of modern society is the obscenely common use of sugar in nondessert foods. Although it's fairly obvious to most people that a glazed doughnut isn't the healthiest choice (10 grams of sugar), a Thai chicken salad from California Pizza Kitchen contains over four times as much sugar (45 grams). Sure, there are additional benefits from eating salad vegetables, but would you have guessed you were eating the equivalent of four doughnuts worth of sweetness by ordering a salad?* Or would you have felt virtuous for ordering a salad and maybe have allowed yourself to sample something from the dessert menu after such a healthy dinner? We'll discuss how to avoid these pitfalls in later chapters, but keep in mind that avoiding sugar doesn't end when you pass up the dessert cart.

What about other sweeteners? Sometimes people ask about more natural or "less processed" sweeteners like honey, agave, and molasses. Other folks want to know about calorie-free sweeteners like stevia and sucralose (Splenda). My answer, to many people's surprise, is to pick whichever one tastes best with what you're eating (even if it's plain old cane sugar) and don't worry about it. The thing about sugar is that no matter what form it comes in, it's still sugar and is not good for you. Moreover, foods that require sweetening (e.g., pastries) usually have enough other unhealthy ingredients that swapping out the sugar isn't going to make a huge difference. Maybe molasses has a little more vitamin D or agave ranks a little lower on the glycemic index (because it has more fructose, similar to high-fructose corn syrup), but that doesn't change the fact that these are still highly concentrated sources of sweetness and should not be eaten in large quantities.

But that doesn't mean you shouldn't eat them at all. There's room for small amounts of sugar in a healthy diet, and it doesn't much mat-

---

*One of the huge benefits of eating fresh, local, and seasonal veggies is that, because they are naturally sweet and filled with flavor, you don't need nearly as much sugary dressing to make them taste good.

Sugar Content of Some Common Food Products

Item	Grams of Sugar
Krispy Kreme original glazed doughnut	10
Luna Bar, berry almond	11
Froot Loops breakfast cereal, ¾ cup	12
Ben & Jerry's vanilla ice cream, cup	16
Starbucks Caffè Latte, 16 ounces	17
Godiva truffles, 2 pieces	17
Subway 6-inch sweet onion teriyaki chicken sandwich	17
Mrs. Fields chocolate chip cookie	19
Tropicana 100% orange juice, 8 ounces	25
Yoplait original yogurt, 6 ounces	27
Craisins dried cranberries, ⅓ cup	29
Vitaminwater, 20 ounces	33
Oscar Mayer Lunchables, crackers, turkey, and American cheese	36
Coca-Cola Classic, 12 ounces	39
Sprinkles Cupcake, red velvet	45
California Pizza Kitchen Thai chicken salad	45
Jamba Juice, blackberry bliss, 16 ounces	49
Odwalla SuperFood, 15 ounces (450 ml)	50
Starbucks Caffè Vanilla Frappuccino, 16 ounces	58

ter where it comes from. Don't forget to keep everything you eat in perspective. You could get hit by a bus tomorrow. Then how virtuous would you feel for ruining your grandmother's famous apple pie recipe by swapping out sugar for Splenda? We all know pie isn't the healthiest thing in the world, but some experiences have more value than nutrition alone. As long as you don't choose experiences over health every single day, those occasional indulgences are not going to kill you.

Artificial sweeteners have other problems as well. Despite their lack of calories, evidence shows that people who use noncaloric sweeteners do not weigh any less than people who don't use them. People tend to think they are being virtuous if they choose lower-calorie foods over higher-calorie foods, but without an obvious benefit, what is the point exactly?

Lack of effectiveness is not my only issue with artificial sweeteners. Some studies have suggested that consuming calorie-free sweeteners enhances a person's appetite and cravings for sweet foods, and this has been proposed as one of the reasons they are not effective at helping people lose weight.

The safety of several of the most popular sugar substitutes has been questioned as well. Though I've never found any of the arguments about the dangers of saccharin (Sweet'N Low) or aspartame (Equal) particularly convincing,* they are relatively recent additions to the human diet, and the long-term consequences for you as an individual remain unknown. So if you really want to cut back on sugar enough to suffer through the taste of these nouveau chemicals, keep in mind that you are essentially volunteering yourself for a long-term human health experiment that may or may not work out in your favor.

In my opinion still the strongest reason to avoid artificial sweeteners is taste. To me there is something innately unsatisfying about the taste of no-calorie sweeteners, and bad-tasting desserts are a paradox of the worst kind. But the assault on your taste buds doesn't stop there. Artificial sweeteners keep your palate accustomed to overly sweet foods (most are hundreds of times sweeter than table sugar), making it more difficult to reacclimate to the taste of real food. So not only do artificial sweeteners ruin your dessert experience; they also ruin your healthy eating experience. Awesome deal, right?

---

* The original studies were flawed, and both sweeteners are officially considered safe for human consumption.

I make one notable exception with these recommendations. Diabetics have a medical condition that prevents them from eating sweet foods that impact blood sugar. This includes cane sugar, honey, agave, molasses, and most other forms of natural sweeteners. The only exception is the stevia plant, which is a natural* calorie-free sweetener that has been used therapeutically for hundreds of years. Stevia has been shown in some cases to reduce hyperglycemia and hypertension in patients with preexisting conditions and is probably the best option for those who cannot tolerate any kind of caloric sweetener. Because the benefits do not exist for nondiabetic patients and, like other calorie-free sweeteners, stevia is still hundreds of times sweeter than sucrose, I do not recommend it except in these specific clinical conditions.

Flour is another food that's high on the not-so-good-for-you list. The refinement process kills most of the nutrients and makes your body digest it so rapidly that it can really mess with your metabolism. Most flour is fortified to add back the lost nutrients, but you're still better off skipping it or at least minimizing how much you eat. Because your body digests it so rapidly, flour is one of those foods that is very important to keep in small portions. The less you eat at one time and the slower you eat it, the better.

Processed meats also appear to be pretty darn bad for you. Though the mechanism that makes them more likely to be associated with cancer and heart disease still isn't exactly clear, it probably has something to do with the smoking and curing processes. Although all cured and processed meats seem to contain some level of carcinogenic compounds† (few processed foods do not), there seem to be higher levels in processed meats that were cured using industrial methods[18] compared

---

* The process of extracting the sweet chemical from the stevia plant has to be done in a lab, so some have questioned why stevia powders can be labeled as "natural." You can grow stevia in your garden and use the raw leaves if you prefer.

† Technically they're called polycyclic aromatic hydrocarbons, or PAHs.

to those cured by more traditional methods in Spain and Portugal.[19] Personally, I find traditionally smoked and cured meats like Italian prosciutto and Spanish jamón ibérico to be exceedingly delicious, and I make room for them in my healthstyle on occasion. I just keep in mind that large quantities could potentially be dangerous, so I keep my portions moderate.

EAT FOOD (AKA THE LARGE PRINT)

I got a little technical in the last few sections in order to satisfy the more skeptical among you, but rest assured that you don't need to know a single detail about saturated fats or insulin metabolism to make perfectly healthy food decisions. The gist of what I just explained is beautifully summarized by Michael Pollan in his book *In Defense of Food*: "Eat food. Mostly plants. Not too much."[20]

We could fight all day (and people do) about what molecular components constitute an "ideal diet," but we already know enough about the foods that promote health and the foodlike products that don't. The overwhelming trend in everything we know about healthy eating is that real foods, the kind that come from the land, air, and sea, are usually good for you. You may need to moderate your portions of some to get maximal satiety with minimal calories, but for the most part as long as you're choosing something one of your pre-twentieth-century ancestors would recognize as food, you're probably on the right track. On the other hand, almost all processed foods, even those labeled "healthy" because some magic nutrients have been added, are more likely to not live up to their claims and may even cause problems down the road.

Believe it or not, all of this is awesome news. Real food is actually much simpler to deal with than all the fancy scientific food invented in the laboratories of food companies. It's fairly easy to recognize, since it hardly ever has a label extolling its health benefits. The ingredients are easier to pronounce. It tastes way better and varies from season to

season, so you never get bored. There are also plenty of real-food options, so if some childhood trauma is preventing you from ever eating
beets again, there are plenty of other healthy, delicious foods to fill in
the blanks. Choosing real food allows you to eat the things you love,
and you always have the option of adding or subtracting based on your
circumstances and even your mood. No arbitrary lists or meal plans for
you. You also have the freedom to tinker with your healthstyle, finding
the ideal fit for your preferences and metabolism. Some people thrive
with more protein, others with more starch. As long as the source is an
unprocessed food, you have nothing else to worry about.

A FOODIST'S PLATE

I've now mentioned portions a few times, and it's something we'll talk
about in more detail later, but it can be helpful to have a visual image

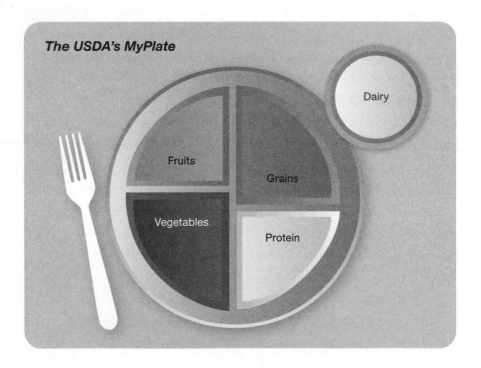

of what an ideal foodist's plate looks like for making the best food decisions. I was actually pleasantly surprised when the U.S. Department of Agriculture (USDA)* came out with its most recent dietary recommendations, which get rid of the antiquated food pyramid and introduce the much simpler MyPlate. But although the new plate structure is helpful, there are still enough flaws in its design to warrant a do-over.

My problems with MyPlate? First, Americans are so confused about the status of fat that I think it needs to be addressed, but you really have to dig through the MyPlate literature to find its out-of-date recommendations. On my Foodist Plate I specify that vegetables should be cooked or prepared with natural, minimally processed fats and oils.

---

* If you think it's odd that the same government agency whose job is to promote the U.S. agriculture industries is telling us what is and isn't healthy to eat, you are not alone. An FDA-sponsored recommendation, without so many obvious conflicts of interest, would make much more sense.

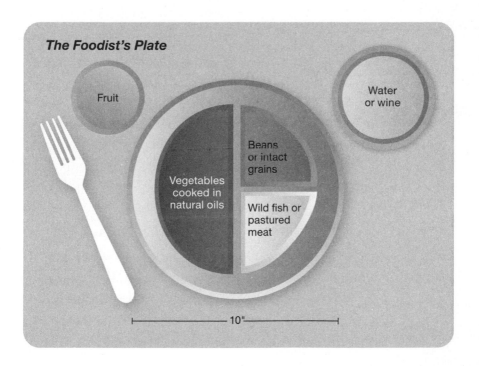

The Foodist's Plate

Fruit

Water or wine

Beans or intact grains

Vegetables cooked in natural oils

Wild fish or pastured meat

10"

Also, I don't think fruit belongs on a dinner plate. I put it on the side to indicate that it should be used for snacks or dessert. The My-Plate proportion of grains is much larger than necessary, and I think beans or lentils are a preferable form of starch. Additionally, "protein" is very vague, so I went ahead and specified the option of wild fish or pastured meats (eggs are a good choice too). I consider dairy optional (sorry U.S. Dairy Council) if you're eating plenty of vegetables, meats, and legumes. If you want to throw some milk, cheese, or butter in there, I have no problem with that, but I don't think it needs its own special section any more than things like nuts and seeds do.

Last, water is what you should be drinking most of the time. Tea and coffee are also perfectly healthy, and wine appears to have some unique health benefits, including reduced risk of heart disease and preserving cognitive function. I'd add that your plate should be about 10 inches in diameter or less. At any given meal there can be deviations from this example, but this is a great place to start if you're revamping your healthstyle.

DON'T FREAK OUT

The last thing I want to add here is that there is no need to freak out about any meal or ingredient. Our biology is amazingly resilient, and if there's one consistent finding in the scientific literature on health and nutrition, it is that long-term dietary patterns are far more important than single foods or temporary deviations from your normal behavior. A splurge In-N-Out burger every now and then, so long as it doesn't happen too regularly, is nothing to be ashamed of.* It is virtually impossible to avoid every carcinogenic molecule lurking in your food, but that doesn't mean you'll get cancer from a single bite. The best any of us can hope for is to minimize our exposure whenever possible (keep-

---

* That's what she said.

ing in mind that there's a good chance we don't know what is and isn't problematic) and try to maintain the healthy activities that seem to fight these diseases like eating fruits and vegetables, avoiding too much sugar, and getting enough exercise.

Similarly, do not be discouraged even if your average meal falls outside the range of what I suggest in my ideal Foodist's Plate. Every meal does not have to be ideal, or even close to it, for you to be healthy and happy. The Foodist Plate is only intended as an aspirational goal for when everything is going right. If you do not have regular access to local, organic foods, do the best with what you have. Eating vegetables and fruits from any source (organic, local, or not) is better than not eating them at all. If wild-caught fish or pastured meats are unavailable in your area or are too expensive to be a regular part of your diet, that doesn't condemn you to a lifetime of disease and excess belly fat. Maybe you'll need to rely a little more on beans and lentils or have to eat farmed and canned fish every now and then.* But you can still eat healthier than the vast majority of Americans and continue to eat the foods you love by simply making an effort to eat more fresh vegetables and fewer processed foods. Upgrading your healthstyle is about figuring out what works for you, regardless of the circumstances you find yourself in.

---

* I've done all this and more while trying to make ends meet through college and graduate school.

PART II

GETTING STARTED

"The distance is nothing; it is only the first step that is difficult."

—MADAME MARIE DU DEFFAND

FIVE

KNOW THY FOOD

Two Weeks of Tracking, Because You're Worth It

"Real knowledge is to know the extent of one's ignorance."
—CONFUCIUS

"Knowledge rests not upon truth alone, but upon error also."
—CARL JUNG

"The wise know their limitations; the foolish do not."
—BENJAMIN HOFF, *THE TAO OF POOH*

Understanding how to eat for health and weight loss is essential for becoming a foodist, but upgrading your healthstyle will be difficult until you know exactly what your current habits looks like. Remember that almost all of your eating is done on autopilot, as a result of unconscious scripts that play out in response to different environmental and internal cues. As a result, most of us are frighteningly unaware of exactly what and how much we're eating.

If you've been on and off of diets for most of your life, you may think you're better at monitoring yourself than most people—you've had a lot more practice, after all. But as we've seen in previous chapters, chronic dieting tends to make us ignore internal cues and lose track of how much we've eaten when we exceed our goals. So contrary to what you might expect, dieters are usually much worse at self-monitoring than other people. Even scarier is that we don't even realize how bad at it we are. The only way to solve these deficiencies is to unleash our inner scientist and, at least for a little while, become data junkies.

A FOODIST'S JOURNAL

Humans are notoriously terrible at recalling what they've eaten. Study after study has demonstrated that we consistently underestimate the amount of "unhealthy" foods we eat and overestimate the "healthy" ones.* We are also awful at judging how much food we eat. For decades scientists believed that overweight individuals did not eat significantly more than normal-weight individuals, because differences were not re-ported on food-frequency questionnaires. However, more careful mea-surements revealed that overweight people do in fact consume more, but consistently underreport how much food they eat. Though at first some scientists assumed this was a personality trait of overweight and obese people (maybe the participants were delusional or simply lying), further research revealed that the overweight are in fact no worse at estimating portion sizes than normal-weight people and do not under-report their food intake intentionally.

The reason for the reporting bias was a mystery until 2006, when research by Brian Wansink and Pierre Chandon showed that, although heavy and normal-weight people are good at guessing the size of small portions, both groups are horrendous at guessing the size of larger por-

---

*Though our perception of what is and isn't healthy is subjective and largely determined by the diet trends of the time, throughout most of the twentieth century people have underestimated their consumption of foods high in fat and sugar and overestimated their intake of vegetables and fruit.

tions. The bigger the portion, the bigger the error, and these miscalculations can result in underestimating calorie content by up to 40 percent. Wansink and Chandon showed that overweight people underreport how much they eat simply because they consume larger portions, and this fact alone explains why they are less aware of how much they're eating.[1]

Given what we know about how environmental triggers impact what and how much we eat (how big are your kitchen plates, exactly?), it stands to reason that any of us can become inadvertent overeaters with the wrong habits or in the wrong environment. This is particularly true of chronic dieters, who are even more susceptible to environmental cues that trigger overeating, and may explain why dieters tend to gain more weight than nondieters over time.

Fortunately, there are plenty of tools that can help us overcome our propensity to delude ourselves about what and how much we eat. The first step in breaking the illusion is collecting accurate information. Just as in the lab, the best way to get good data in the kitchen is to measure, measure, and measure some more. Don't worry, I won't ask you to carry around kitchen scales and measuring cups with you for the rest of your life. But diligently measuring and recording how much you eat for a couple of weeks can be incredibly instructive for determining your optimal healthstyle.

The first thing you'll need is a place to record your entries. I prefer to log my activities in a small notebook I carry in my bag, but if you want to use an iPad or other digital device, feel free. The only requirements are that you can update your journal from anywhere (i.e., it's mobile) and that data entry can occur quickly enough to not be a hindrance in your daily life. A fancy spreadsheet in Google Docs is great, but if you can only access it from a desktop computer and data entry is a pain, then you'll be more likely to forget what you ate and rely on recall rather than specific numbers. Consequently, you will get less reliable information from this exercise. Mobile apps such as MyFitnessPal are another alternative.

When you enter information in your journal, the most important thing is that you are brutally honest. Omit nothing, not even that one pretzel you snagged in the lunchroom off your friend's plate, and do your best to give the most accurate description you can. Include the food item you're eating, how large the portion is, and what sauces and other ingredients are used if applicable. Record the time of day you eat (the times you wake up, fall asleep, and exercise are helpful as well) and if possible how you feel afterward. The more healthstyle data you collect, the better.

It helps to have exact measurements of everything you eat, so a small kitchen scale and/or measuring cups and spoons make this a lot easier. You can even buy special bowls, cups, and other utensils with built-in measurements if you find these easier to use, though they are certainly not necessary. Consider bringing your tools with you to work (or bringing in an extra set) if it's not too embarrassing. If you can't get exact measurements (no, I don't think you should bring your own bowls to Chez Panisse), estimate the volume of your food the best you can by comparing it to common objects like a golf ball, a baseball, a deck of cards, and so on. Take pictures with your cell phone if it helps you keep track.

I realize this may sound a little intense, but you won't have to keep this up forever. Two weeks is my minimum recommendation, and you will find the benefits of putting in this kind of effort early on to be more than worth it. For starters, even though I have not suggested making any dietary changes at this point (we are only documenting your current healthstyle for now), almost everyone who goes through this exercise will lose some weight. Why? For the same reason the control group in every diet study loses weight. This is what I refer to as the quantum effect of dieting: simply measuring your eating habits is enough to alter your behavior at a subconscious level.

We can't help but behave better when we feel like someone is watching us, even if that someone is our future self (or our iPhone). So chances are that during this time you will make healthier choices and serve yourself less food. But weight loss is not the point of this exercise. The practice of keeping a rigorous food journal, even for a short time, has a multitude of benefits. Measuring your food forces you to pay attention to portion sizes. Not only will this prevent you from overeating in the present; it will also teach you to be a better judge of portions in general and help you avoid the pitfall of underestimating the impact of big portion sizes moving forward. For example, you'll learn to eyeball what a half a cup of oats looks like both dry and cooked, and you'll have a better sense of how much wine you really drink at your weekly dinner parties.

Though few of us are born with the skill of judging portion sizes, research has shown that people can get better at it with training. Food journaling will also help you identify your habitual eating patterns and, as a result, help you isolate the triggers, scripts, and rewards that are causing you to eat unconsciously. A detailed journal helps you find bright spots and weaknesses in your healthstyle as well and is something you can turn to anytime you get stuck or feel as though you aren't making the kind of progress you expect. Sometimes you won't notice a patterned behavior or habit until you force yourself to write it down several days in a row. Have a weakness for after-dinner snacks? Maybe you're not eating a satisfying enough meal, or maybe a difficult family situation or school-work procrastination is triggering you to eat more than you need. Could your morning doughnut habit be solved by eating a bigger breakfast at home or moving your workout from evening to morning? Once you clearly see your problems, you can go about finding the best solutions. Last, your two-week food journal gives you your first taste of what it feels like to practice mindful eating, a critical component of upgrading your healthstyle, which we'll discuss in chapter 7.

Sample Foodist's Journal

Monday

11:00 A.M.	½ c. muesli w/ hemp milk, cinnamon
12:30 P.M.	Iced coffee, no cream
4:00 P.M.	Workout
5:00 P.M.	Starving! Spinach feta Peasant Pie
8:00 P.M.	Dinner at Dosa: split Chenai chicken (w/ salad), dahi puri, and lamb curry w/ lemon rice with Kevin
Evening:	2 glasses white wine
Total steps:	15K
Comments:	Late start was a killer, threw off my whole day

Tuesday

8:30 A.M.	½ c. warm muesli, Americano w/ splash of cream
1:00 P.M.	2 scrambled eggs in butter, ½ c. kimchi
4:00 P.M.	Workout
5:30 P.M.	Coconut: water and flesh
7:30 P.M.	Lacinato kale (1 bunch), 4 oz. tempeh, sautéed w/ soy sauce and garlic; 1 very small avocado
Total steps:	14K
Comments:	Dinner was good, but a little too big; felt much better today than yesterday

Wednesday

8:30 A.M.	½ c. warm muesli, Americano w/ splash of cream
11:45 A.M.	Lunch at Plow: roasted kabocha squash salad, arugula, hazelnuts, vinaigrette, asiago; 1 bite of Kevin's egg scramble (tomatoes, spinach, feta); herbal iced tea
2:00 P.M.	Workout
4:00 P.M.	Early Girl tomato
5:30 P.M.	1½ c. homemade popcorn w/ butter, salt
6:30 P.M.	Roasted chicken leg, 5 very small potatoes, mixed green salad w/ tomato, carrot, radish, basil, vinaigrette
Total steps:	13K

Thursday

9:00 A.M.	Workout
11:00 A.M.	Muesli, coffee per usual
3:30 P.M.	½ leftover chicken breast, 4 small potatoes, 2 Early Girl tomatoes
6:30 P.M.	Got roped into 5-course pasta-tasting menu (required whole-table participation); hardly any veggies; hard to track portions, but tried not to get full; had a few dessert bites; wine pairings, about 2½ glasses total
Total steps:	12.5K
Comments:	Dinner not that good; felt like a waste of an indulgence

Friday

7:30 A.M.	Warm muesli, coffee w/ cream
11:30 A.M.	Workout
1:00 P.M.	Half chicken breast plus wing, 2 very small potatoes, mixed green salad w/ carrot, radish, tomato
7:00 P.M.	Sautéed tempeh and radishes, tossed w/ radish greens and avocado, oil, vinegar
Total steps:	11K
Comments:	Good day

Saturday

11:00 A.M.	Coffee w/ cream
12:30 P.M.	Fresh English muffin, butter, poached farm egg, smoked salmon, dry-farmed tomato slices, arugula (homemade w/ farmers market ingredients—epic)
12:45 P.M.	Roseblush apple
3:00 P.M.	Workout
5:00 P.M.	¼ c. trail mix
8:00 P.M.	At party: 2 slices roast beef, 2 (duck?) lettuce cups (mostly veggies), assorted cold vegetables, 3 whiskey punch cocktails; dessert: many raspberries, a few strawberries, 4–5 chocolate bites
Total steps:	13K
Comments:	Should have eaten more dinner food, less sugar

Sunday

10:00 A.M.	2 cappuccino
11:00 A.M.	2 scrambled eggs w/ scallion (cooked in butter), 1 Arkansas Black apple
1:30 P.M.	Organic chicken fajitas, fresh guacamole, tortilla chips (1 c. chips)
6:00 P.M.	1 c. homemade roasted tomato and pepper soup w/ horseradish/chive crème fraîche, pan-roasted brussels sprouts w/ pine nuts, cannellini beans w/ butter, olive oil, parsley, 1 Italian sausage (Whole Foods), 1 glass red wine
Total steps:	10K
Comments:	Felt like too much food today. Full.

LOOKING FOR TRIGGERS

When you begin to notice patterns in your journal, start paying more attention to what you're doing right before these actions occur. Are you at work? In the car? In front of the TV? Are you tired? Bored? Sad? For all habitual behaviors, there is something that is triggering you to do what you do. Your job is to find the cues for all your habits, both good and bad.

The reason for identifying negative triggers is probably obvious to you by now. Once you know the cue that is triggering a particularly fattening habit of yours, you can work on identifying the reward that made the habit stick and devise a new script, so you can replace that habit with a healthier one. But there is value in analyzing good habits as well. Good habits are your bright spots, the activities where you are virtuous without even trying, and these provide valuable insight as to what sort of behaviors are the easiest for you to integrate into your healthstyle. Your bright spots can also help you identify the kinds of cues and rewards that motivate you to act in a healthy way.

IDENTIFYING REWARDS

No habit forms without an associated reward. The problem is that the reward you receive by completing a certain habit is not always immediately apparent and can often be very subtle. Never assume that a reward is obvious. For example, if you have a habit of eating an entire pint of ice cream every Sunday evening during *The Simpsons,* you might think you do it because the ice cream is just so good you can't resist. But this is probably not the case, and it certainly doesn't explain why you eat the entire thing and don't just have a few bites as the packaging recommends.

One thing I've discovered since switching to unprocessed, real food is that most of the things I considered decadent treats in the past really aren't as good as I thought they were. When you start to appreciate that even vegetables can taste amazing, your standards for what is worth eating drastically rise. Also, your palate acclimates to real flavors, and it becomes easy to recognize the overly sweet, salty, and creamy (i.e., fatty) concoctions that pass for indulgence in the industrial food chain. Your mouth starts perceiving these imitations for what they really are: bad for you, without any real taste. These realizations can go a long way toward changing your attitude about certain foods, but they don't necessarily make it any easier to break a bad habit. What they can show you, though, is that you aren't necessarily overeating because this food is so amazing you'll never be able to taste anything like it again. You are eating out of habit, and the reward is likely more psychological than perceptual.

To identify a reward, use a method like the one described by Duhigg in his cookie experiment. In order to figure out why he was eating a cookie every day at 3:30 P.M., he isolated the three parts of his activity that could be the source of his craving: (1) the sugar, (2) the physical act of getting up from his desk and moving around, and (3) socializing with friends. It seemed obvious the reward was the cookie. Don't we eat cookies because they are filled with delicious sugary goodness? To test this, he tried replacing the cookie with a candy bar, but was careful to eliminate another critical part of his habit—the socializing. It turned out the candy bar failed to satisfy his craving, so a sugar fix was not what Duhigg was really after each day at 3:30 P.M.

Similarly, he tested the hypothesis that he was just antsy to get out of his seat and move a little. When he allowed himself this reward (taking a walk) while restricting his sugar and socializing, he learned that physical movement was also not the reason for his daily pilgrimage to the cafeteria. His final hypothesis was that he was motivated by a desire to socialize, which he tested by walking to the cafeteria and chatting with colleagues without actually buying anything to eat. Indeed, this was the only activity that was as satisfying as his original cookie adventure; it seems his elephant wanted to gossip. He used this knowledge to construct a new habit using the same 3:30 P.M. trigger, but instead skipped the cafeteria and chatted with coworkers on his own floor.

Duhigg deconstructed his habit by isolating the three critical components that had the potential to provide the reward. He then selectively eliminated each action while leaving the others intact, so he could test the ability of each to satisfy his craving. Once he identified the reward, he set up a new script for his behavior and was able to alter his habit to achieve his rider's loftier goal of weight loss. Both the elephant and the rider were satisfied with the result, and Duhigg developed a healthier habit.

Changing this one habit enabled Duhigg to lose twelve pounds without any pain or suffering. If this doesn't strike you as remarkable, it should. Duhigg told me his daily cookie was the size of those typically sold at cafeterias, which are not small. A conservative estimate of the calories in one of those cookies is about 350, but a big cookie can easily reach 500 calories. We can therefore calculate that he was eating at least 1,750 extra calories per week in cookies and possibly up to 2,500, almost an entire extra day's worth of food. Just one habit can make a tremendous difference. Although you can't count on all your habit changes having an effect of this magnitude, keep in mind that this was just one healthstyle habit out of dozens that Duhigg was performing each week that were cumulatively affecting his health and body weight.

This is exactly why being a foodist is so powerful. Most of us ignore the dozens of small, mindless activities that habit forces us to do automatically and blame our weak will whenever our cookie craving gets the better of us. But when habits are constructed purposefully, all these little behaviors can have a life-changing impact on how we look and feel. Focusing on eating real food and optimizing your healthstyle with rewarding, healthy habits is much more enjoyable and has a far more positive impact on your quality of life than any restrictive diet could ever pretend to offer.

TAKING INVENTORY

By the time you've finished with two weeks of food journaling, you should have a good idea of where your healthstyle stands. Even if you think you know all your habits, take a minute to skim your journal and look for repeated entries. Anything you've done more than two or three times in two weeks is a potential candidate. Write these down in two columns, one labeled "Healthy" and the other labeled "Could Be Healthier." The goal here is not to judge yourself and feel guilty. The goal is to identify the habits that will be the easiest to move from the latter column to the former column as well as those that will have the largest impact (like Duhigg's 1,750 weekly cookie calories).

For each habit in the "Could Be Healthier" column, attempt to identify the cue and the reward. Put a question mark next to those for which you can't pinpoint either the cue or the reward and pay special attention to these mystery habits over the next couple weeks. Perform experiments like Duhigg's that help you isolate possible rewards and test how well each reward is able to quench your craving. Your ultimate goal is to understand what triggers all of your habits and what your elephant is seeking when it carries out your script. This will give your rider a fighting chance to guide your elephant in a new direction.

Some habits will be easier to rescript than others. Start with those. For instance, eating a pastry for breakfast every day is an easy one, and cutting out this habit could be as effective as Duhigg's cookie elimination. Simply replace it with something healthier and tasty, like eggs, hot muesli with cinnamon, or plain yogurt with fruit. This may require a bit of grocery shopping or waking up five minutes earlier, but it should be fairly easy to reprogram. Most of us sleepwalk through the morning anyway. Start with the easy stuff, and don't bite off more than you can chew. Working on two or three new habits at a time is reasonable, but more will take up too much of your mental resources and leave you too depleted to carry any of your plans through.

EXTENDING BRIGHT SPOTS

Good habits are your bright spots, and these can often be expanded or mimicked to replace some of your "Could Be Healthier" habits. For instance, one reader found that she loved cooking meals from scratch on the weekends, but on weekdays she often made excuses not to and ended up making poorer food choices as a result. Together we analyzed what was preventing her from cooking dinner on weeknights despite her best intentions. The moment of her decision was her cue. Although she thought she was too tired after a long day of work, she realized that what usually prevented her from making dinner was a lack of ingredients and simple meal ideas. She already had the healthy habit of going grocery shopping most weekends, but she usually found recipes beforehand and only shopped with these and snacks in mind. It was less fun for her to plan a week's worth of meals when she was so excited about trying one new recipe.

The solution was to change her shopping strategy and channel her weekend enthusiasm into preparing a few ingredients that could be

How to Make Your Own Muesli— It's Stupid Easy

Muesli is my favorite alternative to traditional breakfast cereal. It's minimally processed, has no added sugar, and when made properly is quite tasty. The only problem is that these are features that food companies hate, because foods that have them are not big sellers. This makes it difficult to find muesli, particularly a high-quality version at a reasonable price.

Luckily, it's stupid easy to make your own muesli. Doing it yourself is also a lot cheaper and lets you customize the mix to your preferences. All you need is some rolled grains (oats or mixed grains work fine) and an assortment of nuts and dried fruits of your choosing—you don't even need a real recipe.

For my personal recipe I use a five-grain cereal that I found at my local market (about $2). I add some roasted and lightly salted mixed nuts, some extra hazelnuts (because I love them), some golden raisins, and some dried currants (about $4 total). It tastes amazing, even better than the expensive stuff I used to buy, and lasts much longer.

I sometimes eat my muesli mixed with a little plain yogurt, but these days I prefer to just pour half a cup of it into a bowl (I leave a measuring cup in the container as a scooper), add some water, and microwave it for 2 minutes. It comes out like the tastiest oatmeal you've ever had. I sprinkle a hefty dose of cinnamon on top and maybe add a splash of unsweetened hemp or almond milk, and it tastes delicious. If you're still acclimating to the lack of sugar in muesli, you can try stirring in a spoonful of peanut butter, low-sugar jam, or honey.

used in several dishes throughout the week. She discovered that as long as she had an idea of what could be eaten as a main course, usually a protein-rich food like roast chicken or simmered beans, then it was easy for her to visualize herself throwing something quickly together after work by adding some vegetables to an ingredient she already had.

All she had to do was to alter her shopping routine to include a single item that could be used as a main course for several days and buy a few extra vegetables that go well with everything (broccoli, kale, and carrots became her go-tos).

Another friend solved a similar problem in a slightly different way. He prefers not to give up any of his weekend time for shopping, but doesn't mind cooking at home on weekdays, since it is usually faster than going out in the city. He opts to do his shopping on Monday nights after work instead, but allows himself to pick up dinner from the Whole Foods deli that night, so he isn't overwhelmed by having to both shop and cook or shop and go out on the same night. Now he can get a decently healthy and tasty meal on Mondays, then have plenty of food to cook for the rest of the week. Weekends he usually eats at restaurants, but his healthy weekday habits have helped him maintain a twenty-five-pound weight loss.

Finding the Courage to Roast a Chicken

I wish I had a dollar for every time I've heard a foodie proclaim that roasting a chicken is the easiest thing in the world and the perfect place for new cooks to start. Please. I can think of at least a hundred things easier to cook than roast chicken, with salad being the undisputed champion (and scrambled eggs the runner-up).

Buying and cooking a whole chicken requires a number of steps that can make a new cook uncomfortable. First you have to know where to get the chicken—and if you want a pastured, antibiotic-free bird (as you should), this isn't always straightforward. To make the purchase you must also be comfortable talking to the butcher, even though there's a good chance you have no idea what you're talking about. You have to be willing and able to deal with raw meat, which makes many people queasy in and of itself. Cooking meat also requires special equipment, such as a meat thermometer and a roasting pan, which newbies might not have access to. So, no, roasting chicken is not the easiest thing on earth. But if you can get over all those things, it really isn't that hard either.

I had a zillion excuses for why it took me so long to roast my first chicken. I think the main one was that a whole chicken just sounds so big, like too much work and too much food. But I was inspired by Ruth Reichl's recipe in her book *Garlic and Sapphires*,[2] so I finally built up the courage to make it happen.

I'm happy to report that I now roast chickens regularly and finally consider them one of the easier dishes in my repertoire. The difference in flavor between a real farm-fresh chicken and the massive "boneless skinless" breasts I grew up eating is truly phenomenal. That alone is reason enough to try the recipe in my opinion.

Here's the slightly easier version of Reichl's recipe I've adapted.

Simple Roast Chicken

1 3- to 4-pound roasting chicken
Chopped fresh herbs
1 to 2 tablespoons butter (optional)
1 lemon (optional)
Salt and pepper
Olive oil

Preheat the oven to 400°F. Remove the bag of innards from inside the cavity if necessary. Rinse the bird with cold water and pat dry with paper towels. Place the chicken, breast side up, in a 9 × 13-inch roasting pan (one with at least 2-inch sides). Remove the excess fat from near the tail and put it under the skin of the breast meat (or use a couple of pats of butter if there isn't enough fat). Season the meat by placing fresh chopped herbs like rosemary or chives under the breast skin with the fat or butter. Put a fork-punctured lemon into the cavity (optional, but recommended). Coat the skin with salt, pepper, and olive oil, and bake for 1 hour or until the temperature reaches 165° in the thigh meat (away from the bone).

Sure it's simple, but I know I'm not the only one intimidated by the idea of buying and cooking an entire chicken.

If you don't know where your bright spots are, turn to your journal and ask yourself when you eat the healthiest food, when you do your grocery shopping, and when you get the most exercise. What are the cues and rewards that help create these situations? Can they be repeated elsewhere or work on a slightly different task? Also pay attention to where you are at these moments, along with who you're with and how you feel. Don't panic if you can't identify many bright spots. Chapters 10–13 offer plenty of tips on how to upgrade breakfast, lunch, and dinner in different settings.

ORDER OF OPERATIONS

Just as important as choosing the right habits to reprogram in the beginning is the order in which you tackle them: if you start by trying to eliminate all the cookies and doughnuts in your life without finding anything to replace them with, you'll basically be putting yourself right back on a deprivation diet and sabotaging your efforts.* In the first few weeks of upgrading your healthstyle your focus should be on eating *more* healthy foods that you enjoy, not cutting stuff out. This will help you create a foundation of healthy habits that gives you something positive to build on.

Summer Tomato reader Patrick Birke is a perfect example of the kind of success that is possible when you get your healthstyle timing right. Patrick's journey started when his first daughter was born in 2009. Wanting to feed her the healthiest food they could find, he and his wife subscribed to a Community Supported Agriculture (CSA) farm share (we'll discuss these more in chapter 6) not far from their home in Minnesota and started making their own baby food. This exposed them to a world of new vegetables, and fresh food became part of their lives. But when their summer share of the CSA ended and they were

---

* Reread chapter 2 if you need a reminder of why this is a bad idea.

left with only meat from the animal CSA they subscribed to through winter, Patrick reached his highest weight ever and realized his diet wasn't yet optimal. The following spring they subscribed again to their vegetable CSA, and Patrick added some exercise to his healthstyle. He made a little progress on his weight, but it wasn't until summer that he was ready to start cutting junk foods out of his diet. By autumn he had lost forty pounds and decided to continue his vegetable CSA through the winter. A year later he had lost more than sixty pounds, and over the next two years he's maintained a sixty-five-pound weight loss.

Would Patrick have had the same success if he attempted to make these changes in a different order? I don't think so. Popular TV shows like *The Biggest Loser* help people lose weight by severely restricting food and implementing strenuous exercise programs. Sadly, weight loss through these methods almost never lasts, and the contestants are notorious for gaining the weight back.* For Patrick, maintaining his weight loss has been easy because he spent the first year developing healthy habits that he actually loves. "Eating healthy has become second nature, and I don't even think about it," he told me. He also explained that he now feels the urge to work out so strongly that it's "almost like an addiction." That doesn't sound like deprivation to me. It sounds like an incredibly effective healthstyle humming away on autopilot. Though a show about people like Patrick would never be dramatic enough to make it on TV, if it did, it would have to be called *The Biggest Winner*.

To achieve success like Patrick's, start your healthstyle upgrade by focusing on *eat more* habits, rather than *eat less* habits. These will make it easier to cut back on less healthy foods in the future. Try eating a healthy breakfast every day and adding more vegetables to lunch and dinner. Over time these habits will reduce your need for willpower by eliminating feelings of deprivation and restriction. Other habits that a

---

* It breaks my heart to think how demoralizing this must be for them.

10 Simple Goals to Get You Started Eating Healthy

1. Eat breakfast

Eating a healthy breakfast is one of the easiest ways to improve your healthstyle. Breakfast is quick and easy to make, and even healthy ones taste great. Start here to automatically improve 30 percent of your daily meals.

2. Buy groceries weekly

Shopping is an essential habit for the obvious reason that to eat better, you need to have better food in your house. Get yourself on a regular, practical shopping schedule, and don't be lazy about it. Use all that willpower you saved up by ditching diets and build a healthy shopping habit.

3. Eat something green at lunch and dinner

This is one of those simple, easy-to-implement changes that gets you in the habit of making healthier choices on a regular basis. You don't need to go all in on salad every time, just try to include something green, even if it's a small side dish. Train yourself to eat those veggies.

4. Eat fish three times a week

Fish is especially healthy, and getting in the practice of having it several times a week is a great habit to develop. When possible, use fish to replace less healthy foods, like processed meats.

5. Limit added sugar to once a week

It's smart to start recognizing foods with added sugar for what they are: dessert. If you're currently eating a lot of sugary foods, start by cutting back gradually, working your way down over time. The important step is that you learn to keep track of how often you eat dessert each week and keep the number in a range that optimizes your health and happiness.

6. Try a new type of vegetable every week

In the foodist spirit of adventure and in the name of nutrient diversity, getting in the habit of trying new vegetables is an excellent way to keep your healthstyle exciting. There's no need to go nuts with this, but trying a new fruit or vegetable every week or so is a great way to develop your foodist palate, particularly if your current diet is limited to a handful of common items.

7. Bring your lunch to work

This isn't going to be feasible for everyone, but if you can swing bringing your lunch to work, even for a few days a week, it can have a tremendous impact on your health and body weight.

8. Cook dinner at home on weekdays

Even I can't bring myself to cook at home every night, but I make an effort to do it every Sunday through Thursday. The more I succeed, the easier it is to control my weight.

9. Carry a water bottle

I drink so much water that it makes me uncomfortable to go out for more than a couple of hours without bringing my own bottle with me. Thirst is often mistaken for hunger, and staying hydrated is an effective way to dampen unconscious eating habits.

10. Embrace NEAT

Most people think of treadmills and dumbbells when they think of exercise, but simply moving more throughout the course of the day (also known as nonexercise activity thermogenesis, or NEAT) can burn more calories than a daily gym trip. To keep tabs on your activity levels, invest in a pedometer or activity tracker,* and make sure you meet your daily goal.

---

* The Fitbit and the Nike+ FuelBand work well.

foodist should develop early include choosing higher-quality foods over those that might be a "better deal,"* eating nutrient-dense foods to help curb cravings, practicing mindful eating, and adding strategic snacking to prevent mealtime overeating.

When you have built up a few healthy habits and are ready to start cutting less healthy foods out, start with those that you care about the least. Remember, you don't need to eliminate every last unhealthy habit you have; our goal is to just make sure that there are more healthy ones than unhealthy ones, so that they balance out in your favor. Work-related bad habits are an obvious place to start, since unhealthy indulgences you make at the office are the least likely to be worthwhile. Are those cheap doughnuts really worth the ten pounds they've added to your waistline? Probably not. Keep in mind that, even though we try to eat delicious foods whenever possible, circumstances sometimes don't leave us with the best of choices. If your office cafeteria only offers mediocre, not so healthy sandwiches and lackluster salads, the salad is the better choice, even if it tastes slightly less good than the sandwich. Save your sandwich indulgence for when you can get your hands on one that's worth it. If your lunch isn't going to be particularly enjoyable in either case, you might as well go with the healthiest thing you can find.

WEIGHING IN

Just as important as tracking your food and activity levels is tracking your body weight. I know this isn't fun, but it is very effective. And with all the cool new wireless and socially integrated scales on the market, it is actually way less painful than it used to be.

Though some health professionals recommend not weighing yourself daily, the scientific research actually makes it clear that tracking your weight

---

* Everyone loves feeling as though they're getting more for less, but in the food realm this philosophy does more harm than good.

is an effective way to help people stick to their eating plans. The scale is more than a simple guilt-o-meter, and the benefits of regular weigh-ins are far more profound. First, although some have argued that body weight fluctuates too much during the course of the day for daily weigh-ins to be meaningful, this isn't true if you weigh yourself at the same time each day in exactly the same outfit. I recommend hopping on the scale butt naked, first thing in the morning, when you're in a fasted state. This will give you the most consistent results and the kind of accuracy you need to make informed decisions about your eating and exercise habits.

Just like your food journal, your daily weight is a valuable data source. For instance, if you know you are able to lose a pound and a half from Monday through Friday if you cook four of five dinners at home, you can compare this to a week when you go out most nights, but do your best to order healthy food and not overeat. Some people discover going out isn't a problem; others find it makes weight loss impossible. The only way you'll know is if you keep track. Similarly, if you have a tendency to overindulge every weekend, you have that number on the scale glaring back at you Monday morning telling you exactly how much damage was done by that hoagie and those curly fries. You can then make the appropriate adjustments (say, allowing yourself only one pancake at breakfast instead of two) until you find the formula that works. Many people find that gaining a little bit of weight back on weekends is inevitable,* but if you can limit it to one pound instead of three you'll see and feel the difference at the end of the year.

Wireless digital scales are particularly useful, because they allow you to track your weight and body fat over time.† They will even plot

---

*Remember that weekends are one of those wonderful things that make life awesome, so it's okay if you don't eat like a saint.

† WiFi body scales like the Fitbit Aria and the Withings scale have great apps. Tracking body fat is less accurate than tracking weight, but it's interesting to watch it change with time.

it out on graphs and allow you to input additional data, like waist size. If you're brave, you can share this information with your friends and make a friendly competition out of the whole thing, which can be a terrific source of motivation. Having this information keeps you honest with yourself and gives you the knowledge you need to understand what is and is not working. It's much more difficult to optimize your healthstyle without this kind of dynamic feedback to help you make better decisions and stay on track.

LET'S GET THIS PARTY STARTED

A powerful corollary to building a long-term healthstyle rather than going on a temporary diet is that your weight-loss journey begins with your next meal, not on Monday after your friend's thirtieth birthday weekend. Indulgent moments are part of life, and there is no point in turning a blind eye or pretending that they don't matter. To become a foodist, you need to get out of the dieter's habit of scheduling good behavior for when it's more convenient. So start your food journal today, or tomorrow at the latest, and don't put it off even if you don't have a single measuring cup in your entire house. We want a snapshot of the real you, not the ultra-well-behaved-and-eats-perfect-serving-sizes you. This isn't a test and it isn't very hard, and the only way to make progress is to jump in with both feet. Don't worry about what your plans are tonight or this weekend—just grab a pen and start collecting data.

Consider this your first step in training to party like a foodist, where you can leave your fear and guilt at the door, because you know you can have a good time without doing irreparable damage. Starting your journal today will be lesson number one in learning to be honest with yourself and not hiding from your weaknesses. Eventually you'll develop a knack for knowing what and how much food you need to feel satisfied without overdoing it. But you'll never get there without acknowledging where you stand. Remember that we're going for *bet-*

ter eating, not perfect eating. And *better* starts with habits. And habits take practice. Your healthstyle doesn't have a pause button, and you won't get the practice you need by ignoring the times when you aren't on your best behavior. These are instructive moments, and foodists must learn to celebrate without giving up on any of their goals (*including* the goal of fun). Life should be awesome, so we should be able to enjoy ourselves without derailing our health or ruining our good time. There's plenty of room for both.

SIX

SHOPPING AND COOKING

A CRASH COURSE IN BECOMING A KITCHEN NINJA

"Gold that buys health can never be ill spent."
—THOMAS DEKKER, *WESTWARD HO*

"My mother gave me a real kick toward cooking, which was that
if I wanted to eat, I'd better know how to do it myself."
—DANIEL CRAIG, ACTOR WHO PLAYED JAMES BOND

"In spite of the cost of living, it's still popular."
—KATHLEEN NORRIS, AMERICAN NOVELIST

Not everyone likes to cook. In fact, few of us even know how—and these days that's not even weird. I feel fortunate that my parents were at least semidecent cooks, and their lingering 1960s hippie ideology kept me away from too many takeout or overprocessed meals growing up. But for some reason this didn't translate into my being able to cook for myself when I went away to college.

I have far too many embarrassing—and hilarious—memories of my freshman attempts at feeding myself. The first time I tried to make pasta, the pot took so long to boil I forgot about it and literally burned water. I was responsible for five or six egg casualties before successfully hard-boiling one (I was terrified that if I took even one bite of an unset egg yolk, I would get salmonella and die, so runny yolks went straight into the trash). After a few months I pretty much gave up on the kitchen and relied almost exclusively on burritos and café salads for sustenance. Even now, with the food revolution in full swing, I talk to adults every day who have no idea how to do anything more than heat things in the microwave. Apparently cooking is no longer viewed as a skill essential for survival, so most of us never bother to learn. This is a serious problem.

If you're shifting a little uncomfortably in your seat right now, re-lax.* I'm not asking you to become Betty Crocker (nor do I think you should ever use her products). And if you are really, truly incapable of cooking even the bare minimum I recommend here, I will give you some alternatives in this chapter. But at the very least I'd like you to consider the possibility before dismissing it completely. The case for becoming moderately proficient in the kitchen is incredibly strong, and I promise to address all your deepest fears and reservations. Remember, I was the anticook myself before I became a foodist. And if I can learn to fend for myself in the kitchen, so can you.

CONTROLLING YOUR DESTINY

I've never found a more reliable way to lose weight and keep it off than cooking at home. The reasons are pretty straightforward: you can

---

* For those of you who already know how to cook and are wondering what all the fuss is about, I would still recommend this chapter. It will give you good ammo for those inevitable conversations with people who believe cooking and eating healthily are too difficult or expensive.

10 Reasons You Hate to Cook (and What to Do About Them)

I don't like the word "hate" and try not to use it. I especially dislike it when it is applied to any kind of food or cooking. Do you really hate asparagus? Or are you just whining about something you haven't bothered to learn to appreciate? Yeah, I thought so.

You don't have to love cooking, but knowing the basics and feeling competent in the kitchen can open a world of opportunity to improve your quality of life. But sure, go ahead and hate it if you want. For the cautiously curious, here are a few of the obstacles that may be preventing you from getting past your pessimism and what to do to get over them.

1. You suck at it

The first thing you need to do is understand the difference between not liking cooking and not liking to be bad at cooking. Big difference. I didn't like being bad at cooking either, but there is a pretty easy solution: learn how. It's much easier than you think.

2. You're slow

I know you're busy. We all have better things to do than slave away over one lousy meal. But when you aren't experienced in the kitchen, the planning, shopping, chopping, cooking, and cleaning can feel as if they take forever. That's because they do.

I can always spot kitchen rookies by how long it takes them to chop an onion (seriously it takes like twenty seconds max). The good news is that with a little practice and some decent knives (see the next reason), you can slash the time you spend making a meal until you barely notice. Ditto for cleaning up. Seriously, put some muscle into it, and it's over in no time.

3. You have crappy knives

I generally don't advise spending money to solve problems, but knives in the kitchen are an exception. Spending $50 on a halfway decent chef's knife can do wonders for your kitchen confidence and efficiency. And you probably already know what an inspiration a shiny new toy can be.

4. You pick complicated recipes

Some of the best meals I've ever eaten had less than five ingredients. If you've never cooked anything in your life, cassoulet shouldn't be the first recipe you try.

Rather than finding a recipe and deciding to cook it, start with an ingredient that is seasonal and you know you enjoy. It's hard to mess up kale and garlic (try Sautéed Kale with Pistachios and Garlic, p. 239). Learn to fly before you jump off a cliff.

5. You choose out-of-season ingredients

The main reason people don't like (_fill in the vegetable_) is that they have only had it from industrial farms that grow foods out of season. I agree, you'd have to be a masochist to like those clones.

Farmers markets and dedicated produce stands are your friends. In-season ingredients taste worlds better than the out-of-season stuff shipped from the opposite hemisphere. Your food doesn't have to be 100 percent local, but at least pick foods that grow in the same season you happen to be living in. This alone could completely change your cooking experience.

6. Your pantry is inadequate

It can be really annoying to flip through a recipe book or food blog and realize that you need to make one or many grocery trips in order to make any dish, because you don't have olive oil, salt, pepper, red wine vinegar, or red chili flakes. A well-stocked pantry and fridge will remove many of the barriers to cooking at home.

7. You cook everything to death

Just because your mom cooked broccoli until it was dark gray and could be eaten by an infant doesn't mean that's how food is supposed to be prepared. Most vegetables cook quickly and taste better when they haven't been boiled beyond recognition. When your vegetables turn bright green in the pan, that's your cue that the cooking is nearly done.

8. You only cook for large groups

Your first cooking forays shouldn't be huge productions. Instead of hosting a big dinner or bringing food to a potluck of thirty people as your cooking debut, start by volunteering to help in the kitchen with someone who knows what he or she is doing. Or make a side dish or a simple one-pot meal for yourself. Practice makes perfect, and you want your first experiences to go smoothly, so your elephant doesn't get scared away.

9. You only cook for special occasions

New cooks don't need any extra pressure in the kitchen. If you're just learning your way around the range, maybe you should hold off on cooking for your Valentine's Day date. It can be stressful to just coordinate a special meal; you don't need the added pressure of possibly ruining a holiday. Start your real kitchen adventures in the privacy of your own home.

10. You don't ask for help

If you are truly new to cooking, you may as well acknowledge that you will be slow and lack the basic skills and intuition of a seasoned chef. You are definitely capable of getting there, but in the meantime make your experience as pleasant as possible by letting others contribute their expertise and knife skills when you want to cook. It is also nice to have an extra pair of hands for cleanup.

control what's in your food and how much you serve yourself. Even in San Francisco, which is as close to foodist heaven as it gets, restaurants still use obscene amounts of (pasture-raised, hormone-free) butter, (cold-pressed, single vintage) olive oil, and other rich foods. The portions are also far larger than any human really needs and therefore require willpower to resist overeating (because, *damn,* that food is good). Eating at home is simpler, and for a foodist's daily habits, simpler is better. Of course, I have absolutely no problem with eating at restaurants occasionally. My social obligations take me out to eat at least once or twice a week (and that's when I'm being good). But if you're eating out every meal, keeping your weight under control is substantially more difficult.

But let's face it, cooking is about more than just your weight. It's a life skill. Even if you're unlikely to ever be stranded on a desert island and need to feed yourself off the land, there are plenty of real-world reasons you'd be better off with a few kitchen skills. For starters, being able to cook for your date is almost as hot as looking great in those jeans. And gender is completely irrelevant on this one—everyone likes to feel taken care of; it's a basic human instinct. So turn on the romance and fire up that stove. Cooking at home is also more efficient than going out. It's faster and costs less, so long as you know what you're doing (don't worry, we'll get to that part in a second). Cooking is also immensely rewarding. There is something innately satisfying about being able to take ingredients and turn them into a nourishing, delicious meal. Being able to feed yourself is one of those basic human skills that no one should be without.

FEAR IS THE PATH TO THE DARK SIDE

I've heard a thousand excuses for why people don't cook more at home. "It takes too long." "I don't like cleaning up." "It's too expensive." "I hate cooking." I know, I've been there. But next time you find yourself cringing at the thought of pulling out a cutting board, remember the wise words of Yoda: "Fear leads to anger, anger leads to hate, and hate leads to suffering." Instead of grumbling about how much you hate to cook, try asking yourself, "What am I really afraid of?"

When you don't know how to handle food, the kitchen can be a scary place. There are fire and sharp objects, and if something goes really badly, you might go hungry. When you aren't proficient with a knife, cutting and chopping can take forever. If you aren't familiar with seasoning, adding flavor requires a recipe. When you haven't learned to judge when a food is "done" cooking, dinner may be ruined. If you make a mistake, you do not know how to fix it. These are not pleasant thoughts.

Cooking, like any art, requires a baseline level of skill. And like any activity that requires some skill, it will not be enjoyable until you are good at it. Fortunately, cooking isn't difficult to learn, and a few simple pointers can get you to this basic proficiency. Yes, it will require some practice, but if you go about it the right way, the learning curve should be relatively painless.

ESSENTIAL GEAR

It doesn't take much to get started eating better at home. Basically, you need the ability to cut stuff up, cook it, and serve it. However, since our goal here is to make this as easy and enjoyable as possible for you, it is worth investing in a few pieces of equipment that drastically improve the quality of your time in the kitchen (and with any luck keep all your fingers attached to your body).

CHOPPING

A good set of knives is the obvious place to start. Kitchen knives aren't just an expensive status symbol. Sure, there are sets that cost more than your first car, but you don't need anything that fancy to get started. One sharp, well-balanced chef's knife will make cutting and chopping food faster, safer, and more fun. A basic chef's knife can be found almost anywhere, retailing for around $50–60, and with proper care and maintenance can last a decade or more.* If you've never had your

---

*Wüsthof and Henkels are two excellent brands.

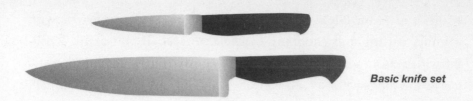

Basic knife set

own good knife, this purchase alone could revolutionize your time in the kitchen.

The only other essential knife you need is a smaller paring knife for more delicate jobs. A chef's knife is great for chopping onions and kale, but can be a little awkward for coring a strawberry or peeling an apple. With these two knives in your arsenal, you should be able to handle any basic recipe, and if you shop around you can probably find them bundled as a set for a small discount. The last thing you'll need is a sharpening steel, the long round poles that often come with knife sets. These help you maintain the sharpness of the blade between uses without grinding down the metal.

If you've invested in good sharp knives, it's also important to have a decent cutting board or two. For cutting vegetables I prefer wooden boards. Look for a cutting board with a fairly large surface area, at least 14 inches long but preferably bigger. (9½ × 13 is common. 11½ × 17½ is ideal.) You're going to want a good amount of space for chopping kale, chard, and other large greens. For omnivores it's nice to have a separate cutting board for handling raw meats. I prefer a plastic board for this task, since it doesn't absorb smells as readily and can go in the dishwasher. It is also handy if your meat board has a gutter carved around the sides to stop any stray juice trickles from getting onto your counter. No matter what kind you choose, be sure to get a board with enough weight, so that it won't be sliding and bouncing around the counter as you chop.*

---

* If you're looking for a well-made but affordable plastic board, OXO makes great products that can be found almost everywhere.

If you're a big fruit eater, you may also consider investing in one additional smaller cutting board that never comes in contact with onions or garlic. No matter how thoroughly you clean your cutting boards, I've found that the flavor of onions and garlic can seep into most foods that are cut on it afterward. Of course, for vegetables this doesn't really matter. But it can be slightly horrifying to take a bite of a melon only to realize you sliced it up in the same spot you mashed garlic and anchovies for that puttanesca sauce on Tuesday night. Blech. Having a separate board for fruit and cheese can prevent such unpleasantries.

The last things you'll need for chopping are a large mixing bowl and a fine mesh strainer or colander for rinsing and straining. The bowl can be used to hold vegetables that have already been cut and to marinate and toss vegetables in dressing. If you get a nice-looking one, it can double as a large salad serving bowl as well. There's no reason this bowl needs to be expensive, but I don't recommend plastic, since it isn't useful for hot vegetables and can sometimes absorb the flavor if it holds food for more than an hour or two. Ceramic, glass, wood, or even aluminum can all make for beautiful and functional mixing bowls. I use my mesh strainer more often than my colander for rinsing and straining (it's particularly nice for straining grains, which may fall through larger holes), but it's convenient to have one with legs as well if you don't mind buying both.

COOKING

Though I wouldn't blame you if your first "cooking" adventures were all just variations on salad (that's certainly how I got started), I presume at some point you will want to eat something warm. Pan sets are another of those kitchen items that can be ridiculously expensive, but really don't need to be. As long as the bottom is decently thick, almost any of the most popular brands of pan sets will serve you well. The advantage of a set is that you'll get all the essentials, including a basic frying pan (this is what you'll use the most), a deeper fry pan with taller sides for larger dishes, a basic pot for boiling, a larger stock pot, lids, and a few bells and whistles like an omelet pan. You can get a decent nonstick set on sale for around $100.

But, wait, doesn't Teflon kill you? There are a lot of rumors and old wives' tales on the Internet, but there is actually very little data that Teflon is dangerous. It is true that if your pan is heated to ridiculous temperatures, the fumes of burning Teflon are not very healthy for small birds,* but for most humans in a normal kitchen setting there is pretty good evidence that nonstick pans are safe to use and won't leech toxic chemicals into your food. They are also much, much easier to clean. If you're a more advanced chef, there are certainly advantages to copper, cast-iron, or even stainless-steel cookware, but your average home cook is likely to find these more frustrating than revolutionary. If you're getting married, feel free to add some fancy copper-bottomed pans to your registry, but they are by no means necessary for a wonderful cooking experience. If a big pan set isn't in your budget, invest in at least one heavy-bottomed frying pan and one pot for boiling. You can add the rest as you go.

You will also need a few utensils for turning foods you're cooking. I highly recommend using 12-inch nylon-tipped tongs for nearly everything, including stir-fries, turning roasts, and tossing salads. Honestly, it's nice to have two pair, if you can splurge on the extra $12.99. That lets you have one for veggies and one for meat or be a little lazier about cleaning. Being tongless is the worst. The other cooking utensils you'll need are one good spatula for eggs and turning more delicate items, a decent ladle for liquids, and a slotted spoon for things like beans. None of these have to be fancy; the nylon ones work great for me.

Last, you'll need at least one good roasting pan. This is the long metal or Pyrex pan with 2- to 3-inch sides that you use in the oven. There are enough life-changing roasting recipes in this book alone to

---

* These were the conditions of the study most cited by the Teflon-will-kill-you crowd.

make a nice roasting pan a worthwhile purchase. If you value the skin on your fingers, you should purchase an oven mitt as well.

EXTRA CREDIT

Once you're ready to go beyond the basics (which honestly shouldn't take very long), there are a few more discretionary items that most people find useful. One is a 2-cup Pyrex measuring cup. As we discussed in chapter 5, knowing how much of something you're using can be helpful. A sturdy measuring cup is also handy for mixing dressings and marinades and can be microwaved if necessary. Similarly, measuring spoons can really come in handy, especially if you start playing around with cuisines that use a lot of spices, like Indian food. If you can find them, I recommend getting measuring spoons that are as narrow as possible (think long and square, as opposed to big and round), so they can reach into tiny jars and containers. You'll thank me later. Consider spending a few dollars on a vegetable scrubbing brush and peeler as well, which can shave a ton of time off your produce-cleaning protocol. If you're a meat eater, you'll also want to invest in a decent meat thermometer. I like the ones that allow you to set an alarm when it reaches a certain temperature, so you're less likely to forget and overcook your meat.

There are a few bigger items that I also recommend for medium-level cooks, including a pressure cooker (for quick beans), a slow cooker (for easy meals), and a hand blender for soups and sauces. I eat enough beans that I consider my pressure cooker indispensable. Canned beans are often flavorless, have a strange texture, and can be, ahem, gas-provoking, but dried beans that have been soaked and cooked on the stove taste amazing and don't cause any digestive issues. The only problem is that cooking beans on the stovetop in a regular pan can take hours, depending on the bean. In a pressure cooker, however, beans cook up in less than twenty minutes, and a single batch can last nearly a week. For $60, it's hard to beat a pressure cooker for kitchen efficiency.

Slow cookers are equally useful, but for the opposite reason. Instead of decreasing cooking time, as their name suggests, slow cookers are perfect for one-pot meals that essentially cook themselves all day while you're at work. They are ideal for large cuts of meat (e.g., pork shoulder) and hearty vegetables, and few things are as comforting during the winter months as coming home to the smell of a delicious, hearty, home-cooked meal. It's enough to domesticate even the most dedicated urban restaurant goer. You can get an excellent slow cooker for $50.

A hand blender (also known as an immersion blender) is another ingenious device that changed the way I work in the kitchen. In the past if I wanted to blend a soup or sauce, a food processor or regular blender were my only options. Since both of these tend to result in big messes and occasional accidents,* using them always seemed too complicated to be worth the extra effort. They are also more expensive. My hand blender changed all this. Now I can submerge the blade directly into the pot I cooked my vegetables in and instantly create a creamy, perfectly smooth soup or sauce. A hand blender is also great for making dips like hummus, and blended foods are now far more likely to appear on my dinner menu.

Pressure cookers, slow cookers, and hand blenders are important, because they enable you to make large batches of food that can be used for several meals throughout the week. This removes some of the biggest barriers to cooking, because it gives you something substantial (e.g., beans, a roast, or a soup) to base subsequent meals around and therefore makes future decisions to eat at home that much easier. This is a good thing. Remember that your elephant is lazy, so you should prioritize tasks that save you future time and effort (i.e., let you be lazier tomorrow). Tricks like these make it far more likely your kitchen time will be rewarding and develop into a habit.

---

*Never fill a blender to the top with hot liquid unless you want a face full of scalding soup.

Since you're now committed to making large batches of food, you'll need a place to store them. It's worth investing in a decent food storage set, whether it's plastic or glass. The Pyrex sets are more expensive but they're sturdier, can be heated, and are potentially safer, since plastics can sometimes leech chemicals into foods. If you don't want to spend a lot of money, feel free to buy the cheap disposable kind. You can reuse them multiple times, but when they get gross or break, you can just toss them out without worrying about the price.

A FOODIST'S PANTRY

Once you have your gear, it's time to focus on your pantry. A well-stocked pantry will enable you to turn almost any random ingredient into a delicious meal, since it can provide flavor, variety, and sometimes even substance to other ingredients. Here are the essentials, plus a few more worth keeping around for good measure.

OLIVE OIL

You'll be cooking pretty much everything in olive oil, so it is important to find a brand you enjoy and can afford in large quantities. I don't recommend buying a superfancy kind for everyday cooking, so any cold-pressed olive oil should do the trick. I do, however, recommend finding a nicer extra-virgin olive oil for dressing salads and drizzling on finished dishes. These come in smaller bottles and are more expensive, but you use less, and the flavor is worth the extra cost.

SALT

Like olive oil, salt is indispensable. Though you've probably seen headlines that salt is the devil's seasoning, the truth is that 75 percent of the sodium consumed in the United States comes from processed foods. If you aren't eating those foods, then salt isn't a problem for you. And if it makes your vegetables tastier (and therefore make you more likely to eat them), I'd argue that using salt is healthier than not.

For a basic kitchen I recommend stocking two kinds of salt, one chunky sea salt that you can grind onto dishes and a carton of plain iodized table salt for adding to boiling water, soups, and other liquid-based dishes. Iodine is an essential nutrient, and unless you eat a lot of seaweed (which I do recommend, but may not be practical for everyone), using the occasional pinch of iodized salt is a good idea. More advanced cooks can experiment with the fancy salts from around the globe.

PEPPER

Yep, you'll need pepper. I recommend getting a grinder with some high-quality whole peppercorns. It'll taste better than the generic pre-ground stuff or even the peppercorns that come with the grinder you bought. Call me a snob, but I usually toss those out, because they don't have any flavor. A cheaper option is the spice aisle of the grocery store, which will sometimes carry good peppercorns with their own disposable grinder built into the container.

VINEGAR

Vinegar is one of those things that can sound unappealing if you haven't had much experience with it, but once you start your kitchen experiments, it will become your secret weapon. Vinegar adds acidity to foods, which your palate translates into a sour taste. This might not sound good on its own, but think about what a squeeze of lemon adds to a lobster tail or a splash of lime juice to guacamole (or cold Mexican beer). A hint of acidity can add a brightness to foods that taste dull or flat and is often the best way to fix a boring soup, sauce, or stir-fry. Different vinegars also impart different character to dishes depending on what they are made from. For instance, I prefer a nutty brown rice vinegar when I'm cooking Japanese food, but for a spring salad vinaigrette, I adore a low-acid red wine vinegar mixed with some fruity extra-virgin olive oil, chopped chives, and a hint of Dijon mustard. Balsamic vinegar is another must, because of its distinctive sweet flavor. It's easy to go crazy with vinegar, but if you're just getting started I recommend some decent balsamic, rice, and red wine vinegars to start. They don't have to break the bank, but don't choose the cheapest stuff in the store either.

STOCK

Having chicken, beef, and vegetable stock in your pantry means that on any day of the week you can have soup for dinner. Stock can also add boatloads of flavor to ordinary vegetable and meat dishes, making you wonder how and when you became such an amazing cook. Though die-hard foodies insist on making their own stock, I've found that no matter how many chicken carcasses I save in my freezer, I never have enough stock around to rely on consistently. Consequently, I keep store-bought chicken and beef stock in my pantry for whenever I don't have the real stuff. My favorite lately is the bouillon paste that comes in little jars. I think the flavor is better than bouillon cubes, and they are easier to store than the big boxes or cans of broth. Remember to refrigerate your paste once you open it.

BEANS AND LENTILS

At any given time I have about half a dozen dry bean varietals in my pantry. I also keep several kinds of lentils for good measure. Beans and lentils are both members of the legume family, since they are fruits that grow in pods. I always make at least one large batch of beans or lentils to supplement my meals throughout the week.

GRAINS

Intact grains are another staple worth stocking in bulk. Of course, I always keep a big container full of my morning muesli (see recipe,

p. 103) and enough rolled grains to make another batch when I run out. I also have an impressive stock of farro, my favorite grain to cook with, and two or three kinds of quinoa (pronounced *keen-wah*)—red and black are my favorite. My rice collection includes containers of short-, medium-, and long-grain brown rice as well as some Japanese haiga rice, which has had the bran polished away but retains the nutritious (and flavorful) germ. Though I use all of these sparingly, I consider them essential components of my foodist pantry.

JARRED TOMATOES

Ironically, tomatoes (my website's namesake) are one of the few vegetables that survive the canning process with a lot of their qualities intact. Because of the presence of bisphenol A (BPA) in the plastic lining of cans, these days I usually opt for jars of tomatoes instead. But regardless of the vehicle, I've come to depend on preserved tomatoes whenever I'm low on fresh ingredients or just feeling as though I need more red foods in my life. Added to meat, vegetables, beans, or all of the above, a jar of tomatoes can turn a few simple ingredients into a full meal.

NUTS

Nuts are one of those miracle ingredients that make almost everything taste better and more satisfying. They even bring an air of elegance to a dish that may otherwise seem a little lackluster. The beauty of nuts is they come in so many different sizes and flavors that they're nearly as useful as herbs for mixing up the taste of a dish. I always have a stock of walnuts, pine nuts, pistachios, pecans, almonds, hazelnuts, and macadamias in my pantry, but your imagination is your limit. Go nuts.

BASIC SPICES

I don't recommend buying one of those giant prefilled spice racks that take up half of your kitchen counter with sad, expired herbs. However, there are a few basic spices worth having at all times. For me these include Vietnamese cinnamon, red chili flakes, coriander, cumin seeds, curry powder, dried oregano, cayenne pepper, paprika, garlic powder, and sesame seeds.

FOODIST PANTRY 2.0

The list above is more than enough to get you started, but veteran foodists will probably want to expand their pantry with a few more esoteric goodies. Here are some items that, although not 100 percent necessary, can really take your cooking to the next level. These will let you dabble in some ethnic cuisines without a complete pantry overhaul. Feel free to add or omit whatever you please from this list. This is just to give you a sense of what I keep in my own pantry to get you started.

SOY SAUCE

There's so much tastiness you can make with soy sauce that it's worth always having a supply in the house. Be careful, though. Soy sauce usually contains gluten. So if you are sensitive, be sure to find the gluten-free kind.

FISH SAUCE

I know it doesn't sound appealing, but fish sauce is a wonderful ingredient that, like soy sauce, adds salty and umami* components to Southeast Asian foods. Thai soups are delicious and easy to make, but you'll need some fish sauce in your pantry.

DASHI

If you like Japanese food, you need to keep some dashi around. Dashi is the delicate bonito- and seaweed-based broth that appears in seemingly

---

* *Umami* describes the savory flavor characteristic of proteins.

every Japanese dish. It's heavenly, and you can't make good Japanese food at home without it. It's fairly easy to find instant dashi in dried pellets. It tastes pretty good, but I prefer the bottles of concentrated dashi from the Japanese market here in the city. You may need to bring a Japanese friend to translate if you want to try and find your own.

COCONUT MILK

Cans of coconut milk are an excellent way to mix up a stir-fry, soup, or sauce, so it's worth keeping a can or two in case you get inspired to make something a little different. These days I can often find the little half cans, which are the perfect size for most dishes. If full-size cans are all that are stocked at a grocer near you, remember to freeze whatever you don't use.

DRIED CHILIES

My dried chili collection is almost as impressive as my bean collection. I have dried dragon peppers, ancho chilies, Thai chilies, cayenne chilies, you name it. Dried chilies have a more complex flavor than fresh chilies, and you can amplify this by toasting them a bit in a pan before using them. If you are among the capsaicin intolerant,* remember that not all peppers are spicy, so even you can benefit from keeping a few in the pantry. I usually dry fresh chilies myself in a low oven during the peak of chili season, but even if you buy predried chilies, they're great to keep around to add depth to any dish.

DRIED MUSHROOMS

Similarly, dried mushrooms have a different flavor from fresh mushrooms and can turn a boring broth or sauce into an amazing one. You don't need a lot. I like to keep a small supply of dried porcini mushrooms for Italian dishes and dried shiitake mushrooms for Chinese

---

* Capsaicin is the active chemical in hot peppers.

cooking. Mushroom broth is also an excellent substitute for beef broth if you're looking to make a recipe vegetarian-friendly.

ANCHOVIES

Another misunderstood ingredient, anchovies are more than just small, salty, tangy little fish. Think of them as a seasoning, like salt or bouillon. Rather than adding a fishy taste, they bring depth, complexity, and of course saltiness to a dish. Italians really know how to use them, so if you'd like to explore what anchovies are capable of, find a good Italian cookbook and enjoy. Trust me, you'll love them.

SARDINES

Sardines are less of a seasoning and more of a main ingredient than anchovies. I keep sardines and other preserved fish like smoked mackerel and trout in my pantry for snack emergencies. I find that a can of sardines is a great source of instant protein when I've been unable to make it to the grocery store and have run out of eggs and yogurt. They're an acquired taste, but delicious. If you're a little squeamish about the idea of fish in a can, look for the boneless, skinless sardines. They're a little less alien for first-timers.

PARMESAN CHEESE

Forget about those green cans of processed goop and go directly to the cheese aisle for a slab of fresh parmesan. Like so many other items on this list, you should think of parmesan cheese less like a single entity and more like a seasoning to enhance an already excellent dish. Parmesan is another way to get that salty, umami flavor into drab meals, and just a couple of slides across the cheese grater can transform meat and vegetable dishes alike. A block of parmesan lasts virtually forever in the fridge (small mold patches can be scraped off and the rest of the cheese is still good), and you can even use the rind as flavoring in broths and soups.

PRESERVED LEMONS

Though not as easy to find as the rest of the items listed here, preserved lemons are one of those ingredients that can trick everyone
into thinking you're a brilliant chef. Like anchovies, they bring a
tangy, salty flavor, but their added spices also create a rich complexity. Use them like a condiment in soups and stir-fries, and on fish and
meat dishes, and be amazed. There are many great resources online
to make your own if you can't find any in your town. Store them in
the fridge.

CAPERS

Capers are another way to fancy up a dish without much effort. They're
easy enough to store that I always have some in the pantry or fridge,
and they've been known to save the day on multiple occasions.

OLIVES

Although expensive olives are nice if you can get them, I find that
it never hurts to keep a jar of pitted kalamata olives in the pantry
for olive emergencies. They happen. If you have tomatoes, garlic,
anchovies, capers, olives, and chili flakes around, you always have a
puttanesca sauce available for dinner. What more could you ask for,
really?

EXPANDED SPICES

Chinese five spice, turmeric, smoked paprika, star anise, cardamom,
mustard seeds, and ground cloves are all spices I cannot live without.
Though I don't do it every day, once a week or so I like to make a
dish inspired by some of my favorite ethnic cuisines—Chinese, Indian,
Japanese, Thai, or Vietnamese. Of course, these kind of kitchen experiments aren't a requirement, but they can make your time in front of the
stove more fun and less monotonous.

ESSENTIAL GROCERIES

A stocked pantry is half the battle in building a foodist's healthstyle, but to make tasty meals you'll also need a few fresh grocery items in your fridge at all times. Most of these store well, so if you pick them up every week or two, you're in business. Once you've got these basics, you're ready to start shopping for dinner.

SMALL ONIONS

I rarely buy the big yellow onions (unless I'm making soup, chili, or something similar), but I always have some more delicate onions on hand. There are lots of options to choose from, including shallots, leeks, green onions (scallions), cipollini, ramps, and chives. Unlike their big yellow or red cousins, these have mild flavor and will not overpower a dish or make you cry when you cut them. I rotate through my different options depending on the season. Spring is my favorite time for onions of all denominations.

GARLIC

I don't use a ton of garlic, because too much of it can mask the subtle flavors of the delicious ingredients I buy. But I always have garlic in the house, and I use it almost every day. One clove can absolutely transform a bunch of kale until even kids and teenagers are begging for more. I'm not picky about my garlic; whatever you can find will probably work just fine. Just make sure it's fresh.

LEMONS OR LIMES

The finishing touch of a dish is often what turns it from something good into something great. Sometimes this is a sprinkle of good sea salt or a drizzle of fancy olive oil. But oftentimes it takes a squeeze of lemon or lime juice to get the flavors perfectly balanced. They store well in the fridge, so it's worth picking up a lemon or lime on most of your shopping adventures.

PARSLEY

I don't know when exactly parsley got relegated to garnish status, but it's a tragedy that must be remedied. Flat-leaf, Italian parsley is the most versatile herb I've ever found. Its flavor is fresh and bright, and just a handful of chopped parsley makes any dish taste better. Another bonus is that, unlike some of the more delicate leafy herbs, parsley stores incredibly well in the refrigerator for well over a week. It's the best.

FRESH HERBS

For all other fresh herbs I use a different strategy. Since a little goes a long way, I usually only pick one or two to have in my kitchen each week (in addition to parsley). Which I use depends on the other foods I'm buying. For example, Mexican food thrives with cilantro and oregano. French vegetables are beautiful with thyme. Roasted meats and potatoes go best with rosemary. Mint is wonderful on Vietnamese and Moroccan food. Basil makes almost everything taste amazing. Experiment. Fresh herbs can change the way you approach cooking.

EGGS

Eggs are my number one go-to easy meal or snack. Scramble some up with those green onions we mentioned earlier for a quick two-minute breakfast or lunch. Add an egg to anything to make it more substantial and extra tasty. Boil some eggs and bring them to work for a filling, satisfying snack. I adore eggs. And, no, they do not cause heart disease.

PLAIN YOGURT

Though I go in and out of my yogurt phases, I think it is a great grocery item to keep around for a quick, filling snack. It's great for breakfast with a little muesli and cinnamon. Plain yogurt is also a wonderful condiment and garnish for dishes that can be a quick substitute for sour cream or crème fraîche. Just don't get the sugary fruit (or vanilla) kind that is often closer to dessert than a healthy snack.

CONDIMENTS

My fridge is never without mustard (for salad dressings and marinades), tahini (sesame paste that makes vegetables taste amazing), a tube of tomato paste, and kimchi (spicy fermented cabbage) or sauerkraut (nonspicy fermented cabbage). Though there are a few other miscellaneous condiments in my fridge, these are the ones I find indispensable.

THE PRICE IS RIGHT

Now is as good a time as any to address the biggest misconception people have about cooking healthy foods: price.

Healthy food is affordable, and I am living proof. I developed my foodist healthstyle while living as a grad student in San Francisco, one of the most expensive food cities in the country. The cost of living there is so high that I was spending over 30 percent of my monthly salary on rent alone, without including utilities, transportation, laundry, or any of the other major expenses of city living. During this time I did the bulk of my grocery shopping (not just occasional special items, but literally breakfast, lunch, and dinner) at the Ferry Plaza Farmers Market—known to be one of the more expensive markets in the city—and opted for heirloom and organic ingredients whenever possible.

How did I do it? I was selective with my purchases. I focused on vegetables and made fruits (which really are more expensive) my splurge items. I relied heavily on beans, lentils, grains, and eggs, saving pastured meats and wild-caught fish for weekends or as a supplement to other satisfying ingredients. Most important, I cooked at home far more often than going out.

The reality is that even organic vegetables are affordable at a farmers market. I've never seen a bunch of kale cost over $2, even from the most high-profile organic farms in the Bay Area. And this isn't unique to San Francisco. A report published in 2011 by the Northeast Organic Farming Association of Vermont showed that national farmers market prices are competitive with and often lower than supermarket prices for conventional produce. For organic produce, farmers markets were cheaper than supermarkets in every instance.[1] Though the results surprised a lot of people, they shouldn't have.

Supermarkets are middlemen. Cutting them out and buying direct from farmers means lower prices. What's remarkable is that it often means higher-quality produce as well. Since local farms are more likely to be selling fresher, seasonal produce, it will taste better than anything shipped last week from the other side of the globe. Farmers market produce is one of those things that everyone assumes costs more than it really does, which would have made my organic broccoli an excellent ploy for fooling people on *The Price Is Right*.

But if farmers market food is so affordable, how did it get the reputation for being an elitist tool of oppression? The answer is fruit. Shoppers rarely buy vegetables, and most people who attempt to increase their fruit and vegetable intake for the sake of health do so by eating more fruit, and only more fruit. Vegetables are an afterthought and are usually ignored. Though I haven't seen any data on why this is the case, I'd wager that it is a combination of ignorance (what the heck is kohlrabi anyway?) and a lack of cooking skills (Mom, do you know what "blanch" means?). Fruit is easy to eat and full of sugar. Consequently, everybody loves it. Vegetables are a little trickier and more mysterious, and I'm guessing this is why most of us don't bother.

Fruit at the farmers market is unlike anything at the supermarket. It's fragrant, it's soft, it's heavy, it's ripe, it's seasonal, it's delicious. All these things make it expensive to transport, because even with all the extra packaging required to keep it safe,* there are still a good number of casualties in each crop.† Supermarket fruit, in contrast, is designed for mass production and transport. It's often picked green and ripened later with gas. It's usually lightweight and hard as a rock to prevent bruising. Industrial fruits are also harvested year-round, whether they are in season or not. This brings down the cost substantially, but as you can imagine it pretty much annihilates any flavor the fruit may have possessed. To combat this reality industrial fruit growers select for breeds higher in sugar, hoping the sweetness will mask the lack of flavor and complexity. These fruits can sometimes taste okay, but they pale in comparison to the luscious seasonal gems I find at my local market. For these reasons, I think the pricing of fruits at farmers markets is fair. That doesn't mean I can always afford it, but it does mean that when I do decide to take home a sweet O'Henry peach or two, I cherish every juicy drop.

The problem ordinary supermarket shoppers have when they walk into a farmers market and see the price of peaches is that they have no idea why these fruits are so much more valuable (and cost so much more) than anything they could get at the grocery store. They then take a look at the tags on the strawberries and melons and conclude that farmers markets are for elitist yuppies, but not for regular folks on a budget trying to feed their family well. What they don't see is that the humble zucchini sitting next to those peaches are sweet, crisp, and rich in earthy complexity, and that they will completely change the way those shoppers think about summer squash and have them looking forward to zucchini season for years to come. They also won't realize that they can get enough to feed their entire family for a few dollars, and even the kids might start liking vegetables if they shop here regularly.

---

*Ka-ching!

† Ka-ching! Ka-ching!

I have seen the graphs showing that it costs more than seven times as much to get your calories from carrots than from potato chips, but I've never understood why this comparison was relevant. Obesity is most prevalent among the poorest socioeconomic classes. Clearly getting enough calories isn't what most people—even very poor people—need to worry about. Not to mention the fact that obesity itself comes with a tremendous price tag. It seems to me that the most important question is how much nutrition we get per dollar, and by this measure a foodist's diet wins every time. Moreover, vegetables and other nutrient-rich, calorie-poor foods tend to take up more volume on a plate, and research has shown volume to be one of the most important factors for feeling satisfied after a meal. I'm not making the case that everyone has the time or ability to shop for and cook healthy food (though I will help you as much as I can with this book), and I think it's a tragedy that for so many people it's easier to get foodlike products than real food in this country. But I do want to make it clear that most of us can afford to eat healthy, delicious food if we care enough to make it happen.

SEASONAL SHOPPING

Keeping my rant about farmers market prices in mind, when you're deciding where to buy your food, it's important to keep perspective on why foodists make the choices they do. Life should be awesome, and investing a little extra time and money into getting high-quality, seasonal vegetables that actually taste good should be one of your top priorities. We're talking about more than a financial transaction here— this is about quality of life. The quality of *your* life. It's about how delicious food, feeling well, and looking amazing contribute to your state of mind. Never forget that you'll only achieve your goals if your elephant is happy. This means that the more shopping and eating experiences you enjoy every day, the easier it will be to succeed.

FARMERS MARKETS

Ideally you will find a local farmers market that you can call your own. I understand that for many of you it isn't feasible to go to the market every single week for groceries, but even going on occasion can deepen your appreciation for truly excellent agricultural products and where your food comes from. Farmers markets are popping up all over the world at an incredible rate, so there's a good chance there is one near you even if you do not know about it. Localharvest.org is a fantastic resource to find the markets closest to you.

COMMUNITY SUPPORTED AGRICULTURE

Community Supported Agriculture (CSA) is a wonderful alternative if time or location is keeping you from a farmers market. CSA is a kind of subscription to local farms. In exchange for a precommitment to buy from a particular farm, the farm will offer weekly or monthly produce or agricultural products at a discounted rate and often even deliver them to your house. Though a CSA subscription may not be able to cover all of your grocery needs, it will definitely get you a step closer to local, seasonal eating.

Like farmers markets, CSAs can vary greatly in quality and how they operate. I recommend finding a few options in your area using localharvest.org and then looking for reviews to see what might work best for you. The biggest complaint I've heard about CSAs is that during certain months the offerings can get repetitive. Some people like this (if you're into canning and food preservation, this is your ticket), and some people don't, so you should make sure that any CSA you pick is a good fit for you. For those of you in colder climates, CSAs can be a good answer to the dearth of produce during winter months. For instance, Foxtail Farms in Wisconsin stores some of its summer produce to supplement its CSA box during the winter. Pretty clever, right?

PRODUCE MARKETS

Don't worry, there's plenty of great produce out there even if you can't buy direct from farms. I've never been in a town that didn't have at least one dedicated produce market. Though all their offerings might not be organic, smaller establishments are still likely to get better-quality produce than giant supermarkets. They are often more affordable as well. If you can't find one in your immediate neighborhood, check Google or browse any ethnic neighborhoods that may be in your town. Cultures that still rely on real food can usually find it somewhere, even in the smallest U.S. cities.

SUPERMARKETS

Although supermarkets have their uses, I generally consider them a last resort for buying produce. The number one reason for this is that the industrial produce purchased by supermarkets is bred for durability, mass production, and ease of transport, not for taste. As a result, the food is often flavorless and doesn't do you any favors in your quest to eat more vegetables. Giant industrial farms are also more likely to use genetically modified (GMO) foods and large quantities of pesticides. Even if you do find yourself in a supermarket for produce, I'd recommend getting as many organic options as possible to avoid pesticide exposure, which has been linked to Parkinson's disease, several cancers, and other nasty things. As you'll likely find, supermarket organics won't taste much better than conventional produce, but will be substantially more expensive. This is why farmers markets are the better option.

My only exception to the supermarket rule is Whole Foods. Though it isn't perfect, Whole Foods certainly makes an effort to get higher-quality produce, and I've sometimes seen food from the same local farmers I buy from at the farmers market. The downside of shopping at Whole Foods for produce is that it is more expensive, but for the increase in quality (and therefore the likelihood of your sticking to your healthstyle plan) I think the extra cost is worth it. Whole Foods also has fantastic seafood and meat departments and is very good about labeling where the animal products come from; the company seems to sincerely care about animal welfare and sustainability, which translates into higher-quality food. The good news is that outside of the produce and meat departments most Whole Foods products are competitively priced with other stores. There are some exceptions, but I've found I can get great deals on real, nutritious foods if I look for them. The bulk bins are particularly useful if price is a concern.

As a general rule the healthiest, least processed foods can be found along the perimeter of the grocery store. This is where you'll find the vegetables and fruits, fish, meats, eggs, and other natural foods. There will be some impostors out there as well,* so don't forget to check labels carefully. The main exceptions to the perimeter rule are dried goods, including grains, nuts, beans, and lentils; bottled and canned condiments, like olive oil, vinegar, jarred tomatoes, and anchovies; and many of the other pantry items mentioned above. You'll have to go aisle spelunking to get those. I'm also a fan of frozen fruits and vegetables. Once you branch out from these sections, you're treading on dangerous territory.

If for some reason you do find the need to browse some of the packaged food options (it happens), a few rules of thumb should help you separate the heirloom farro from the industrial chaff. Food manufacturers bank on your lazy elephant being on autopilot, and rightfully so. Front-of-package health claims are well known to increase food sales, so of course those big, brightly colored "Trans Fat Free!" proclamations are more about marketing than health. Foodists avoid this sales trap by ignoring every claim on the front packaging and turning immediately to the back or side of the package in search of the one thing that really matters when you're buying packaged foods: the ingredients.

---

* Loaves of industrial bread can easily contain over thirty ingredients. And I don't know how they get so much weird stuff in fruity yogurts (or should I call them frootie yogurts?).

At least forty synonyms for sugar are commonly used in packaged foods, and if any of these appear in the first three to five ingredients listed on the back,* I'm probably not going to buy it. If you need a confirmation, you can glance over at the Nutrition Facts and check how much sugar is present in a serving. If it's 10 grams or more, whatever you're holding is probably not your best choice. If it has more than 15 grams of sugar, you can go ahead and call it dessert. For comparison, a Krispy Kreme glazed doughnut contains about 10 grams of sugar.

Be suspicious of any packaged food that has more than five ingredients. And if any of the ingredients contain numbers or acronyms or

---

* They are often *most* of the first three to five ingredients.

42 Code Words for Sugar

brown rice syrup	coconut palm sugar	brown sugar
cane sugar	beet sugar	pear juice
maltodextrin	fruit juice	concentrate
corn-syrup solids	concentrate	maple syrup
refiner's syrup	maltose	simple syrup
evaporated cane juice	treacle	muscavado
sucrose	agave nectar	corn syrup
glucose	molasses	dextrose
evaporated cane juice crystals	inverted sugar	grape sugar
caramel	palm sugar	sweetened condensed milk
dextrin	date sugar	barley malt
golden syrup	gum syrup	corn sweetener
dried oat syrup	carob syrup	dehydrated cane juice
crystalline fructose	high-fructose corn syrup	sorghum syrup
malt syrup	honey	

How to Find Real Food at the Supermarket

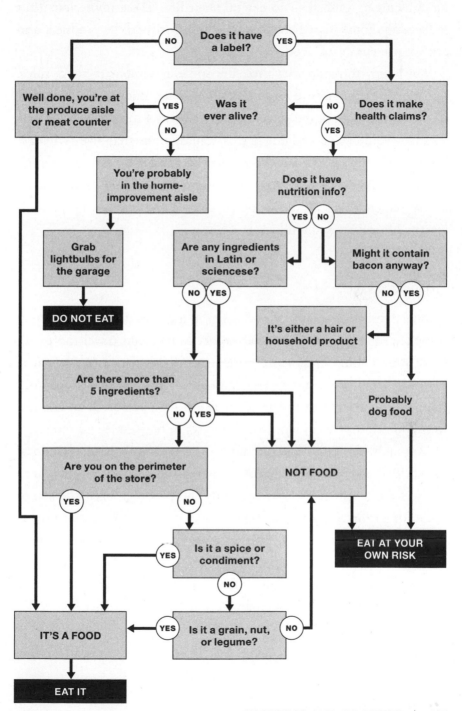

sound overly sciencey,* remember that they are probably there for the manufacturing process or to extend shelf life. These mysterious (but sadly ubiquitous) ingredients are hallmarks of foodlike products and are not present in real food.

I'm happy to report that there are some exceptions to these rules. I've seen a few progressive food companies that proudly put their ingredients on the front of the packaging (personally I think this should be an FDA requirement) and others that contain more than five extremely healthy ingredients. This is wonderful, and I hope more companies follow suit, as consumers start to demand it. That said, focusing on the ingredient list is always the best way to know whether a product is worthy of being called food.

THE ALTERNATIVE

I understand that no amount of begging and pleading from me will convince some of you to cook at home. Maybe you travel too often, work bizarre hours, or don't have adequate kitchen facilities. Or maybe my arguments above just weren't enough to get you to change your mind. If you're willing to brave it, there are a few resources for you lost souls, but most of them will cost you extra in both time and money.

Arguably the safest bet for daily premade meals is at your local health-food store with a deli or prepared-food section. When in a pinch, I'll often swing by Whole Foods and pick up a roast chicken or something from the salad bar. Personally, I think I make better-tasting food at home, but what I pick up is usually passable and finding something healthy and satisfying is relatively easy.

Though it may be difficult, a few healthy restaurants can also be a feasible option for those who aren't able to cook for themselves. I'll

---

* Never eat anything that's been "hydrogenated," even if the packaging claims it is trans fat free.

cover restaurant selection and ordering in chapter 12, but keep in mind that if restaurants are your default food stop, you'll have to be exceptionally diligent in selecting meals and watching portions.

KEEPING PERSPECTIVE

It's unfortunate that sourcing real food has become such a difficult task in industrial societies, and it's important to understand that perfect eating won't always be an option. Do your best to eat well, as often as you can, but don't let yourself become a victim of circumstance. Remember that it's better to eat vegetables, even if they aren't local and organic, than to not eat vegetables at all. Everyone's healthstyle will take a different path, so don't be discouraged if it takes a few weeks before you can consistently integrate healthier foods into your diet. A healthstyle upgrade doesn't happen overnight, and even seemingly small new healthy behaviors bring you a few steps closer to your goal.

SEVEN

ZEN AND THE ART OF MINDFUL EATING

"The problem with the future is that it keeps turning into the present."
—*CALVIN AND HOBBES*

"There's nothing like biting off more than you can chew,
and then chewing anyway."
—MARK BURNETT, PRODUCER OF *SURVIVOR*

Whenever people tell me they eat healthy but still can't lose weight, I ask them if they have tried chewing. After an awkward silence I elaborate and ask if they've heard of mindful eating. At this point most people just continue to stare back at me blankly, wondering what on earth I'm talking about and whether there's a chance I've traded in my lab coat for some New Age crystals and incense.

No, I'm not a hippie. Far from it, in fact. But I do think that just about everyone could benefit from adopting some principles from the Buddhist practice of mindfulness, particularly when it comes to eating habits. "Mindfulness" is just another word for "awareness," and being aware of what and how you eat can have a tremendous impact on both the quantity and quality of the foods you choose. There is a wealth of scientific evidence that eating quickly, not chewing thoroughly, and not paying attention to what and how much you consume can result in substantial overeating. Even healthy foods can cause you to gain weight if you eat too fast or eat enough of them. Though sometimes this mindlessness can be used in your favor (as we discussed in chapter 3), more often than not mindless eating leaves you exposed to dozens, if not hundreds, of subtle cues that trigger you to eat more than you intend. Just as important, eating mindfully helps you appreciate and enjoy your food more, leaving you satisfied with less.

YOU ARE HOW YOU EAT

Have you ever put down your fork for a minute at a restaurant or social event and just watched people eat? It's horrifying, particularly in this country, where we are notorious for gobbling our food. No sooner is a huge mouthful of food shoved into our face than we start poking around the plate for another giant bite, as if the fate of the world were dependent on finishing this meal as quickly as possible. If the fork happens to fill up before we're done chewing, we hurry up and swallow to make room for the next one. An idle fork is the devil's playground. I've seen grown men (you know who you are) put down three pieces of pizza in under five minutes. Even in my own home I've seen half chickens disappear before I can even smooth my napkin onto my lap. Sometimes I wonder why choking isn't contending with heart disease as the leading cause of death in twenty-first-century America.

There has been plenty of speculation regarding why we eat so much more and so much faster than we used to. Some blame the distraction of television and electronic devices; others point their fingers at the deterioration of our hereditary food cultures. I've even heard people blame their siblings and parents for fostering dinner-table rivalries for the last scoop of mashed potatoes. Personally, I blame my own fast eating habits on what for a long time I considered my eating "efficiency." I'm a busy person and have always prided myself on doing things quickly, effectively, and as goal-orientedly as possible. If I could multitask, better still. What I had to train myself to understand is that when it comes to eating, efficiency is not the highest virtue.

Quick eating almost always results in overeating. This is because your brain is not focused on the eating process, but on the goal of filling your stomach. Unfortunately, a full stomach does not automatically create satiety in the brain, which is the ultimate place fullness is perceived. The satisfaction you feel from finishing a meal is only sensed after the culmination of sensory cues and signals indicate that a meal is over. Some of these cues are internal, such as spending time chewing, tasting, and swallowing. Others are external, like seeing an empty plate or noticing a restless dining partner. Only after about twenty minutes will you actually be able to tell if your belly is full or not,* but if you've been stuffing your face the entire time, it is already too late.

How much you eat can easily trump the quality of your food, if you take in enough calories. You've probably heard of the movie *Super Size Me,* in which Morgan Spurlock eats every meal at McDonald's for a month, says yes whenever the cashier offers to supersize his meal, and consequently gains a bunch of weight and develops a slew of nasty health problems. It's an interesting flick, but a few years later James Painter, a professor at Eastern Illinois University, made a similar documentary called *Portion Size Me,* in which he demonstrates that the grossly unhealthy food wasn't necessarily the problem in Spurlock's experiment.

In *Portion Size Me,* Painter had two college students eat every meal at a fast-food restaurant for thirty days. The difference was that the students were only permitted to eat food portions that were appropriate for their body size (one was a small female, the other a larger male). During *Portion Size Me* the students both lost a small but noticeable amount of

---

*This is because our perception of fullness is dependent on a handful of satiety hormones that must be activated (or deactivated) before they can be detected in the brain.

weight and saw improvements in cholesterol and other blood markers, despite all the refined carbs and trans fats they consumed during the course of the film. Eating better food certainly makes eating smaller portions easier* and can improve your health for other reasons, but never underestimate the value of simply eating less for controlling weight and, therefore, getting healthy.

Eating quickly is a particularly effective way to lose track of portions and accidentally overeat. Though the results from research have yielded mixed results,† most studies confirm a link between faster eating speeds and greater risk of obesity.[1] Moreover, intervention trials that retrained overweight individuals to eat slower and more mindfully have been shown to help people lose weight and improve metabolic parameters.[2] Whether it's a plate of salmon and vegetables or a Reese's peanut butter cup, there is definitely a wrong way to eat it.

MIND OVER FATTER

The good news is that mindless eating habits and fast eating can be overcome with practice. The bad news is that, like most bad habits, it is difficult to change your behavior without concerted effort. But if you're committed to the practice, mindfulness does become easier and you'll learn to enjoy your food more and naturally eat less.††

Mindfulness is difficult by its very nature. Sure, if you're aware you're shoveling food into your face, you can consciously slow down and focus on chewing. But since you're likely eating quickly precisely

---

* Ultimately healthy food is more satisfying and will help kill your cravings.

† This is likely due to the large individual differences between people in their response to different foods. Remember that we are all different, so one study will never tell you what works best for you personally.

†† Protip: This is a great place to start using that extra willpower you saved up by ditching your dieting habit.

because your mind is elsewhere, how can you be aware enough to stop yourself? If you are aware, aren't you already acting more mindfully? It's another one of those accursed catch-22s.

The key to developing mindful eating habits is to consciously set up triggers that remind you that you're supposed to be paying more attention to your eating behavior. For example, starting to stab a bite of food with your fork is a defined action that occurs several times throughout your meal. For me, this action is now a trigger that forces me to ask myself if there's already food in my mouth. If there is, I am reminded to set my fork down again and focus on chewing instead. It's amazing how well this works. In this situation, the reward I receive for following through on the habit I've scripted (putting down my fork) is getting to appreciate and enjoy the bite of food already in my mouth. This is actually incredibly satisfying. It's amazing how much of our meals we miss out on by greedily stabbing for our next bite of food when we already have food in our mouths that we're completely ignoring. A secondary reward for following through with this habit is being conscious enough to know when I've had enough to eat and not getting overly stuffed and feeling uncomfortable after my meal.

There are dozens of little tricks you can develop by just spending some time thinking about the actions you go through during a meal. You can then use these to program self-checks on your behavior. For instance, setting the table can remind you to fill a glass of water and drink half of it before starting your meal. Smoothing your napkin on your lap is an opportunity to take a deep breath and reflect that you are about to eat and you should remember to eat mindfully and appreciate your food. If remembering to take a mindful pause is difficult for you, as it is for me, you can use technology to send yourself a helpful ping. When first developing my mindful habits, I set up a recurring event in the Reminders application on my iPhone with notifications reminding me to "chew twenty-five times" before lunch (12:00 P.M.) and dinner (6:00 P.M.). Counting your chews is one of the most effective ways to

18 Tips to Eat More Slowly and Mindfully

1. Practice

Eating quickly is a habit that needs to be broken. Make a point to practice mindful eating by scheduling it into your day. Write it in your calendar, leave notes on your fridge, and send yourself reminders before meals until your new habits become automatic.

2. Chew twenty-five times

Chewing is probably the simplest and most effective way to develop the habit of eating mindfully. There used to be an entire dieting movement, led by the late Horace Fletcher, based on the idea that chewing more helped you eat less. Though Fletcher took this idea a little far (and was arguably a little crazy), there is reliable scientific data that extra chewing results in less overall food intake.

You might think that you chew your food, but there's a good chance you are swallowing a lot of it whole. Take smaller bites and chew your food thoroughly. Notice the texture of what you are eating and appreciate what it adds to your meal. This is something I need to remind myself of directly before I eat, so I keep this on my to-do list. Once the habit develops, you will feel uncomfortable swallowing large, unchewed hunks of food.* I recommend twenty-five chews per bite, but likely anything over twenty chews will provide a benefit. The most important part is that you choose a number and count your chews until you reach it. The number itself is less consequential.

3. Put down your fork

The classic recommendation to put down your fork (or sandwich) between bites has stuck around for one simple reason: it works. When we are not eating mindfully, our hands go into shoveling mode; our fork is primed with another bite almost instantly after popping the last one in our mouth. Putting your fork down forces you to relax a bit and focus on chewing what you already have.

---

* This is actually the reward for your chewing habit—I told you they were subtle.

4. Drink

Another way you can force yourself to slow down is to consciously sip your drink throughout your meal. This requires you to put your fork down, chew, and swallow before eating more. It also adds liquid to your stomach and can help you feel more full. Water is a perfect choice, but even sipping wine can slow down your meal (though it may decrease your inhibition when the dessert menu gets passed around).

5. Feed yourself with your nondominant hand

Making things more difficult is a great way to force yourself to pay attention to what you're doing. One simple way to do this is to force yourself to eat with your nondominant hand, which for 90 percent of us is our left hand. It might be too much to do this for every meal, but trying it for breakfast and snacks is a good place to start. Be careful, though; if you get too good at it, you can slip back into your mindless habits.

6. Eat everything with chopsticks for a week

Even if you grew up with chopsticks as your primary utensil, you've probably never used them to eat a sandwich or a bag of chips. I once heard a story about a local tech company that asked a bunch of its employees to use chopsticks exclusively for a week as a mindfulness exercise. Although weight loss was not the goal, everyone in the office lost weight and several reported life-changing realizations as a result of the project.

One person dropped his morning bagel habit when he realized that the chopsticks prevented him from experiencing the part of the ritual that he enjoyed the most. Apparently the taste of the bagel was not as appealing as the act of rippling the doughy bread apart with his hands. Once he realized that actually *eating* the bagel wasn't important to him, he decided to give it up.

7. Take your first bite with your eyes closed

I once went to a restaurant where the entire dining experience, including being seated at the table, occurred in the pitch dark. The idea was to focus exclusively on the experience of eating, without the distraction of vision. Unfortunately, the food at this restaurant was terrible, and focusing on it only made this point more obvious. But it was a good lesson, and I was certainly not tempted to overeat as a result. Eating all of your meals in the dark or even with your eyes closed is not very practical, but taking the time to taste your first bite with your full attention can help you eat the rest of your meal more mindfully. Focus on all the flavors in your mouth and how they interact as well as the smells and textures. This will help you both appreciate your food and eat more slowly.

8. Eat with other slow eaters

We all have an unconscious tendency to imitate people we are near. If you are dining with ferocious eaters, you might find yourself mimicking their bad habit and eating quickly just to keep up. To train yourself to eat slower, try finding slow eaters to influence you instead. If your rapid dining partner happens to be your spouse,* try asking politely if he or she wouldn't mind enjoying the meal with you by taking it a little slower. I've had nothing but positive responses to such requests.

9. Try to identify every ingredient in your meal

Trying to taste and identify all the different ingredients in your meal is another great way to focus on the present moment and eat more mindfully. This is particularly fun at restaurants, when you didn't make the food yourself. Check your answers by conferring with the waitstaff or asking to see the menu again. An added bonus of this technique is it can also help you become more creative in the kitchen.

10. Use a plate

It may sound obvious, but eating out of a bag is not a very mindful practice. Get in the habit of placing even small snacks and desserts on a plate before you eat them. This will force you to acknowledge exactly what and how much you will be eating.

---

* Welcome to my world.

11. Sit at a table

Once your food is on a plate, you may as well go the extra mile and sit at a table. Sitting at a table to eat tells your brain you are having a meal. If you eat while running errands or standing at a counter, you can quickly lose track of how much you've eaten. Even if you've eaten a fair amount of food while standing, you may still feel as though you haven't had a meal and want to eat more later. Formalizing your dining experience can help draw your attention to your food and your eating habits.

12. Remove distractions

Put away your phone, turn off the TV, step away from the computer, put down your magazine, hide your kids, hide your wife. If you are doing something else, you are not paying attention to the food you are putting into your mouth. I know you are busy and want to multitask, but resist the urge for fifteen minutes and eat a real meal. I admit I'm bad at this one, but I always eat less if I go off-line while I eat.

13. Eat in silence

Although going through an entire meal in pure silence may be a bit much for most of us, designating the first three to five minutes of a meal for quiet and mindful practice can be an effective strategy. Alternately, you can use a single meal each day (like breakfast) to eat without extraneous sounds.

14. Serve small portions

A clean plate is an incredibly powerful cue that a meal is finished. For this reason, large portion sizes often lead to overeating simply because of our tendency to eat what is in front of us. Serve yourself smaller portions as a reminder to take your time and savor each bite. Use small plates, so your brain doesn't perceive the portions as skimpy.

15. Have a conversation

You only have one mouth, and if you are using it to talk, it's really difficult to shove food into it. Though this is the opposite of eating in silence, enjoying a meal with friends and having a great conversation is a fantastic opportunity to slow down your meal. Just remember to chew, so your mindfulness doesn't get thrown completely out the window.

16. Don't eat when you're starving

Nothing makes us more likely to eat quickly than being famished. We may try to eat at regular intervals, but sooner or later circumstances get the better of us, and we end up hungrier than we should be. I always carry almonds or other nuts around with me for times like this, and I eat exactly ten nuts to tide me over for an hour or so. After about fifteen or twenty minutes, my hunger subsides enough for me to regain control of my eating speed.

17. Dim the lights

Research has shown that people eat more in rooms with brighter lights. Set your dinner mood by dimming the lights or lighting candles. This will induce an inner calmness and make it easier to slow down. On the flip side, be careful when eating under bright fluorescent lights, as they can spur frantic overeating.

18. Play mellow music

Slow, mellow music can also help set an appropriate eating pace. Miles Davis's *Kind of Blue* is one of my favorite dinner albums. However, this trick only works if the music is truly slower than your natural, silent eating pace. If your music is any faster, you may experience the opposite effect.

slow down and eat less, and simply requiring yourself to reach a certain number is an effective way many people have been able to control their weight. Try it. It works.

Being mindful of your eating habits is about more than just slowing down. When we're hungry or even just on autopilot (i.e., most of the time), we have a tendency to think we want foods that are decadent and our eyes tend to be bigger than our stomachs. When you see a kind of food you've liked in past, like those amazing bacon- and cheddar-filled potato skins your grandma used to make, it's easy to focus on how tasty you remember them being and not how horrible you'll feel if you put down half a dozen of them before your next meeting. Even worse, if you happen to be at the buffet of your hotel and not at grandma's house, it's easy to forget that the potato skins you're gorging yourself on don't actually even taste that good; they only vaguely remind you of something you once enjoyed. When you're hungry or blinded by memories, it's easy to forget health goals and load up on what sounds delicious. So when you are filling up your plate (or ordering something you'll regret), it's worth pausing and asking yourself not just how these will taste, but how they'll make you feel later.

I'm at the point in my foodist healthstyle where, when I see a cheap, greasy doughnut or bizarrely shiny diner food, I don't see something tasty that I wish I could eat. I've trained myself to see a stomachache, a foggy head, and a big pile of regret. Thanks to this habit alone—thinking about how I'll feel rather than how the food might taste—eating cheap greasy food isn't even tempting to me anymore. Of course, good, high-quality food that happens to be rich and heavy is still very tempting. But I know that if food is high quality, I will only feel gross if I eat too much of it, which is true of anything. Small amounts are fine and every bit as rewarding as I expect them to be, and by practicing mindful eating habits I've learned to stop when I've had enough.

The difference between the two situations is that I make a value-based decision when I eat high-quality foods, whether they are "healthy" or not, and my choices are never mindless. I am fully aware when I am choosing a food for pleasure at the expense of health, and I make certain that it's worth it. I minimize the damage by eating slowly and mindfully, appreciating every last succulent calorie, and am far more satisfied with a few bites than if I ate an entire plate of a less indulgent substitute. For a foodist, making smart food decisions is easy and awesome.

5 Things to Consider Before Eating Something Naughty

Sometimes foods are super unhealthy, but that doesn't mean you shouldn't eat them. Life should be awesome, and the purpose of food should be to optimize the quality of yours. Food is delicious, it makes you healthy, and it brings you closer to friends and loved ones. At any given meal, I try my best to maximize each of these goals. And if it falls short in one, I try to make up for it in another.

Inevitably, there are situations in which the best option is not particularly obvious. For example, how important is it to eat healthy on vacation? Consider dessert. By no stretch of the imagination do we need dessert to live, and if we are being honest with ourselves most of the time we probably shouldn't eat it. But sometimes (er, often) we want to anyway.

Ideally, you should get your healthstyle to a place where you can occasionally go a little wild without it significantly impacting your health goals. But getting there takes practice and a healthy dose of self-awareness.

Here are five questions to help you make the right decision before letting loose.

1. What else have you eaten today? This week?

To be able to indulge occasionally, you need to understand what "occasionally" really means. Depending on your body size and activity levels, you can get away with maybe one or two treats a week. If you find yourself giving in once or more a day, it may be time to reevaluate your definition of "special occasion."

2. Have you been to the gym?

Using the gym to justify a bad diet is a losing battle. But if you do eat a few too many quickly digesting calories, it's much better that they go to fuel your muscles rather than your waistline. I've found that some of my best runs at the gym are on birthday-cake days at the lab.

3. Will you be drinking later?

Alcohol fuels weight gain in a number of ways. Sugary drinks add hundreds of calories to your day and should be considered an indulgence in their own right. Alcohol also has a way of convincing you to opt for late-night burritos and greasy weekend brunches. If you're heading out with friends later, you might want to skip the after-dinner cheesecake.

4. Are you trying to lose weight?

Believe it or not, asking yourself your health goals before you eat something can really help you make better decisions. I don't recommend strict diets when trying to improve your healthstyle, but if you still have weight to lose, desserts and heavy meals won't make your life any easier. If you'd still like to drop some pounds, it pays to be picky with your indulgences.

5. Is it worth it? Really?

One of the best things about avoiding diets is you have the freedom to fit your favorite foods into your life. But one of the downsides is that you need to be able to make good choices for yourself, which isn't always easy. It can be very tempting to consider every cupcake that is brought to the office a special occasion and lose track of the truly valuable indulgences that actually make your life better. Birthdays, anniversaries, and meals at great restaurants are things you will remember for your entire life. Junk food at the office is rarely more than an excuse to avoid work for another half hour. Be honest with yourself about the true value of a food before inviting it into your life.

Don't expect to become a more mindful eater overnight. As I mentioned earlier, mindfulness can be very tough to develop and has certainly been one of the most difficult transitions for me personally. If you're having trouble learning to eat slowly and making more intuitive food decisions, it may help to read about and practice mindfulness outside the food setting, to develop a more mindful life in general.

Mindfulness and meditation have been scientifically proven to benefit their practitioners with things like stress reduction, better focus, stronger personal relationships, and greater well-being overall.

Personally, I've found that being more mindful has helped me get more done at work, because I'm able to spend more time writing and reading scientific journals rather than jumping back and forth between e-mail, Twitter, Facebook, and my calendar. As a result, I finish my work faster and have more time to work out, cook, and spend time with my family, and this has dramatically reduced the stress I feel in connection with these things. Though mindfulness and meditation are often associated with Buddhism, mindful practice does not need to be tied to any religion. Think of it more as the gym for your brain.

THE PSYCHOLOGY OF GOOD TASTE

If you've never tasted a tomato that was so delicious it caused you to abandon a career in neuroscience and launch a food website, I can totally sympathize. I was twenty-six years old before I had my farmers market epiphany and had already lived in the northern California Bay Area (arguably the mecca for local, seasonal food) for nine years. It even took me several years after this experience to truly appreciate that all broccoli and eggplant are not created equal.

When you've spent the majority of your life eating industrial fruits, vegetables, and meats, it's hard to understand how a crazy foodist like me can get so excited about a salad, since the only ones you've ever had could barely be choked down with half a bottle of ranch dressing. There's even a good chance that you don't believe your palate can adapt to eating vegetables or unfamiliar foods at this point in your life. Food preferences and picky eating are deeply personal and can be so ingrained into your psyche as to feel nearly impossible to eradicate. But I've seen countless people (myself included) overcome even their deepest food aversions by developing a foodist's mindset.

Gateway Vegetables

My Story as a Born-Again Foodist

Summer Tomato reader Cheryl-Ann Roberge was a lifelong vegetable hater until one fateful afternoon in July. Her story is not unusual, but it is incredibly inspiring. She tells the story best, so I'll let Cheryl-Ann take it from here.

BY CHERYL-ANN ROBERGE

If you had told teenage me that I would one day be a vegetable lover, spice fanatic, and adventurous eater, I would have sent my canned ravioli flying toward your face. My name is Cheryl-Ann Roberge, I reside in Seattle, and I am a born-again foodist. This is my story.

The 1990s were an underwhelming time in my food life. Eggs were one of the few things I enjoyed eating that didn't come from a box or can. Even at a young age I tried to pick all of the oregano out of my spaghetti. I hated fruit and veggies. I tolerated apples and canned vegetables when required. At age seventeen, I proudly declared that I would never learn how to cook and that I would live solely on canned ravioli. It was simple: I didn't like anything that had real flavor.

Epiphany

Two years into my "adult life," I was existing on a steady diet of Easy Mac and cafeteria food. Vegetables were the most difficult for me. But, ironically, veggies were also the key that would open the door to foods I would never have been interested in otherwise.

I went on about my business of eating meat with noodles or meat with rice or meat with bread, and I was pretty happy with the rotation. I worked in the dorm cafeteria circuit at the university I attended in Milwaukee, Wisconsin, and I liked telling people I was a lunch lady.

On a hot July day, my world was changed. A special picnic for new student prospects was being served outdoors, and I was scheduled to work it. The picnic served food much different from the typical cafeteria fare. After the new students had been served, the cafeteria workers were given a break for a meal together. I loaded my plate with a burger and whichever pasta salad I knew I wouldn't eat much of.

I made my way to the grill and found it covered with a vegetable medley that I'd never seen served before. I kept walking. Mike, the chef, called me back and stuck veggie-filled tongs toward me.

"I don't do veggies, Mike," I said.

"These are different," he explained. He was excited that he'd been allowed to make food he thought tasted good. Mike had once opened his own restaurant, but failed and ended up as a chef at the cafeteria, where creativity was always superseded by budget. This was his banner day.

I declined once more before he gave the overhaul speech that broke me down. He lowered juicy, grill-marked asparagus, onion, zucchini, and squash onto my plate as I shot him a look of disinterest. The veggies were cooked very simply, tossed with oil, salt, and pepper and flung onto the grill. I'd never had anything like this before.

I didn't come away with a huge affinity for onions that time, but I had my first ever delightful experience with something I'd always found disgusting. I suddenly loved the squash and zucchini and thought asparagus was okay too.

Mike told me that I'd made his day. I raved for a week. My whole idea of food turned upside down, and it was just the beginning of a ten-year revolution. I've since learned to like onions, spinach, fish, shellfish, beets, and strawberries. After discovering sushi, wasabi became my gateway into loving spicy food, which I'd never been able to tolerate.

My journey hasn't ended. Last fall I took my first trip to Italy, where I discovered cantaloupe served alongside dinner entrees. I had always been lukewarm about the fruit, but something about having light, juicy melon after a slice of delicious lasagna made me appreciate its sweetness in a way I never had before. Now my least favorite fruit salad element has become a favorite.

It is difficult to express to you just how surprising and lovely these realizations can be. I live for them, and I try every new food I can. I plea-bargain with other picky eaters I meet. I pester them to try new things. I invite them over for dinner and try to introduce them to something they'd never otherwise try.

Why Should You Try and Try Again?

As children, most of us are naturally averse to beer, coffee, and wine. A sip might be granted by a grandpa wearing a grin, which of course is followed by a grimace from the grandchild. So how do most of us end up liking all three beverages despite the horrible trials we go through?

Practice, exposure, and repetition are the keys to comfort. I expanded my taste in music the same way. I started listening to any music I could get my hands on and, as with food, I started having mini music epiphanies too. Consider this: Why did most of us enjoy listening to the radio when we were children? We knew the songs, and they were comforting, like canned ravioli. How do country music haters end up enjoying Neko Case or Ryan Adams? It's fresh and it didn't come out of a can. You get the point.

A Simple Request

As a born-again foodist, I sit here in Seattle writing to you, Picky Eater. I'm late to work, because I care that much about your palate. I want you too to discover the pleasure of new foods. It has changed my life and given me unforgettable experiences with old friends and new.

As a bonus, it's easier to get out and exercise, because I'm not so weighed down by the processed junk food that I used to love. And my waistline is trim now.

Change your ways for those last two reasons if you must, but try new foods because they will eventually taste good and the rest will follow. Just don't expect it all to happen overnight.

Chances are there are foods you love now that you hated as a kid. But how many foods do you still avoid just because *you think* you don't like them? Young palates struggle with things like mustard, onions, and asparagus and instead prefer blander, less intense flavors. But as adults we sometimes cling to these preferences without ever stopping to question the value or meaning of our opinions. But when it comes down to it, what joy is there in being a picky eater?

It is true that taste is subjective, but I've never heard a convincing argument that it's better to dislike a food than to like it. It is certainly more fun to like things, and it is often far more convenient. Just try getting a serious chef to make a signature dish without onions. It isn't easy. But how can you learn to like a food if you don't like the taste?

It turns out that most of the time we decide what we like before we bother to experience it,* and this prejudice clouds our perception of what we actually encounter. This effect of perception bias has been demonstrated repeatedly in psychology experiments in which food color and taste have been manipulated. To see this for yourself, use food coloring to alter the appearance of several bowls of lemon Jell-O and have your friends guess which flavors they are tasting. Very few will say they taste lemon unless the color is still yellow. Most of us taste what we expect to taste, not what we actually experience.

The psychology of taste is further complicated by our natural aversion to things that are new or different from what we are expecting. In these cases the unfamiliarity and strangeness of the food makes us slightly uncomfortable, and we interpret this feeling as a personal dislike. However, this reaction reflects the food's uniqueness rather than its true character. Our tendency to dislike and often hate things that extend beyond our perceptual comfort zones is explored by Malcolm Gladwell in *Blink: The Power of Thinking Without Thinking*.[3] He argues that we make snap judgments about everything we encounter based on prior experience. And although this ability can sometimes help us make wise decisions, it can also explain why pilot testing can't predict the success of new-concept TV shows like *Seinfeld*. Gladwell's book shows us that it's common for our first impressions to be wrong.

Knowing about this bias can help you overcome aversions to foods you think you don't like and even learn to love them. The first step is deciding that there is value in enjoying a food you currently do not enjoy.

---

*Another example of mindlessness.

I'm not saying you need to develop an appreciation for canned peas,* but most fresh, natural whole foods are worth rediscovering for both taste and culture. The second step is persevering in trying the rejected food until you find it prepared in a way you like. This process is not as bad as it sounds, since there is a good chance that the reason you did not like a food in the first place is that what you were served as a child was either canned, frozen, or of industrial (low) quality. Since peaches and plums taste completely different when you get them in season at the farmers market, doesn't it stand to reason that the same is true for green beans, broccoli, and beets? Also, with each new venture your taste will become more acclimated to the flavor and your aversion will dissipate.

Fine dining is a fantastic opportunity to explore foods you haven't enjoyed in the past. I was finally won over on brussels sprouts (my most hated of all vegetables) after a spectacular meal in San Francisco. I learned how to adapt a similar recipe at home and now consider them one of my absolute favorite autumn ingredients. Even if a certain food doesn't end up on your favorites list, learning to at least enjoy it in a casual way will enrich your life and help you develop an appreciation for new and unique experiences.

IT'S A TEXTURE THING

Taste is the sensation we usually associate with food, but picky eaters can be just as fixated on texture as flavor. Ask people who don't like mushrooms or eggplant what turns them off and they are just as likely (if not more likely) to say the food is "slimy" or "mushy" as they are to complain about how it tastes.

Of course, texture is important. It is the essential difference between fresh and stale popcorn and between the springy crunch of a fresh grilled shrimp and the rubbery give of an overboiled one. But for

---

* Gross.

How to Make Brussels Sprouts That Aren't Gross

This is the recipe that finally made me love brussels sprouts. Bacon makes anything taste good, but these days I appreciate the sprouts even without it.

Buy the freshest sprouts you can get your hands on (hint: they're in season in autumn), preferably from your local farmers market. Like any vegetable, the fresher it is, the tastier and more nutritious it will be. I usually buy a pound or so. The smaller they are, the sweeter and less bitter they taste.

The secret is to halve and blanch the sprouts before cooking them with other ingredients. This helps them cook through and gets rid of the nasty, bitter taste that can be so characteristic of brussels sprouts. The other trick is to balance the remaining bitter flavor with an acid like lemon juice or red wine vinegar. Oh, and did I mention bacon? I prefer to purchase my bacon from a local butcher. Get two slices, but for a larger batch of sprouts increase it to three.

This recipe is delicious with either walnuts, pine nuts, or hazelnuts. If you decide on hazelnuts, try them toasted. I like to bake them in the oven (350°F) until the skins start to turn dark and crack, about 10 to 15 minutes. I then roll them in a paper towel or plastic wrap to separate the skins from the nuts. Don't worry if all the skins don't come off; they'll still taste good.

Brussels sprouts pair beautifully with almost any protein. Pork, chicken, and fish work especially well.

Pan-Roasted Brussels Sprouts with Bacon
SERVES 3 TO 4

1 pound brussels sprouts, cleaned and halved
1 cipollini onion (or shallot or leek)
½ cup walnuts or hazelnuts
2 slices bacon
1 tablespoon butter (preferably from grass-fed cows)
Sea salt and pepper, to taste
1 tablespoon fresh oregano leaves, finely chopped
1 tablespoon red wine vinegar *or* lemon juice

To blanch the brussels sprouts, bring water to a boil in a medium saucepan and add a few pinches of salt. When the water comes to a rolling boil, add the sprouts and set a kitchen timer for 5 minutes. Important: do not rely on yourself to remember, as overcooking at this stage will ruin your dish. Boil the sprouts exactly 5 minutes, rinse with cold water, drain, and set aside.

In the meantime, chop the onion and nuts. Stack the bacon and slice into ½-inch pieces. Heat a large sauté pan on medium heat and add the bacon pieces. Allow the bacon to cook about 4 to 5 minutes, until the fat starts to render in the pan. Add the nuts and stir. If you are using cipollini onions or shallots, add those too (wait if you are using leeks).

Cook the nuts and bacon until the bacon is almost done; then add the butter. You can add leeks at this point. When leeks just begin to soften (about 1 minute), add the sprouts, sea salt, and pepper.

Stir the sprouts and turn most of them so the cut faces are down. I strongly recommend using tongs for this. After about 2 minutes, stir the sprouts and sprinkle on the oregano. Continue to cook, stirring every 2 minutes or so until the faces of the sprouts are all browned and onions begin to caramelize, 8 to 10 minutes. In the last 3 or 4 minutes, add the vinegar or lemon juice. This step is essential to cut any last bit of bitterness remaining in the sprouts. Use the taste test to determine precise cooking time (depending on the size of the sprouts).

most picky eaters, the issue is rarely a matter of cooking preference. In the human mind, texture is easily associated with other, nonedible substances that often look, sound, or smell gross. A picky eater who doesn't like a specific texture will often describe the food as feeling like brains, snot, rubber, or other things most of us would agree are unappetizing. Once an association like this is made, the idea can overpower any pleasurable experience that might come from the food.

One way to address this is to form a new association. One of my readers told me he was able to overcome the "dead tongue" feeling of raw fish in sushi when a friend suggested he think of it as lunch meat instead. Though sushi and lunch meat have little in common, this small shift in perception was enough for him to become an avid sushi lover. To implement this on your own, try to think of a food you enjoy with a texture similar to one you don't like. For instance, instead of associating a tomato with snot (I lost track of the number of people who have told me this), try pudding, egg yolk, or a fruit smoothie. If your brain can only come up with gross things, try asking a friend for help.

Another useful technique is to try the offending food in a new setting. An important part of the sushi story is that the person was on vacation in Mexico when he decided to try the raw fish again. When many things are unfamiliar, the strangeness of a particular food texture is less noticeable than it would be if it were the only new thing you were confronting. In another example, a mother cured her child of picky eating by taking him on a trip around the world. The new cultures and environments were enough for her nine-year-old to feel comfortable stepping out of his normal habits and becoming more adventurous.

Indeed, embracing a sense of adventure is very important. Whenever the jet-setting child was nervous about a new food, his mother said she could hear him repeat to himself, "I just have to try it." And no one forced him to eat anything. Repeated brief exposure to something new is sometimes enough for a person to get over the unfamiliar component, which is often the main reason for the aversion in the first place. Almost everyone can learn to like something new if they are persistent enough.

A related approach is to try a food cooked in a new way. I've helped several people overcome an aversion to eggplant that they had attributed to texture by roasting it without much oil. Sautéing can often make eggplant oily and slimy, but roasting gives it a more chewy texture. Once these people realize they enjoy the flavor of the food in this new format, the slimy version is suddenly not so bad.

To some extent, aversion to specific food textures is embedded in Western cultures. In contrast, the Chinese culture embraces food texture as a unique element completely distinct from taste. In Chinese cuisine (the real stuff, not fast-food Chinese), ingredients are frequently added solely for texture, such as jellyfish and sea cucumber. They have little flavor on their own, but add a springy crunch to a dish that is considered a delicacy. Westerners can learn from this approach and develop a more open mind when trying new foods. When you focus on the texture in food not as something you are being subjected to but as a unique and interesting experience to be appreciated, it can break those unpleasant associations and help you enjoy what a less adventurous palate would struggle with.

If none of these works for you, there is always the boot-camp method. One reader explained to me how his son overcame his strong aversion to tomatoes and mushrooms in Marine Corps basic training. After a day of intense training, the recruits were taken into the mess hall, given a plate of food, and told they had five minutes to eat it— the drill sergeant would sometimes count down the final seconds. No other food was available to the recruits, so anything skipped meant less calories and energy for tomorrow. "The recruits ate what was put in front of them or went hungry," he said, so his son tried not to think about it* and forced himself to choke down everything. It wasn't until after he left basic that he realized he was over his food aversions.

Although real, clinical food aversions do exist that can cause people and even babies to gag and vomit in response to certain food textures, most of us can get over texture issues if we want. Persistence, an adventurous spirit, and a few psychological tricks can go a long way toward helping you enjoy new foods.

---

*Sometimes mindlessness has its benefits.

PICKY EATERS VERSUS FOODISTS

It is far more fun to be an adventurous eater than a picky eater, but that doesn't mean you should eat everything that's put in front of you. Always remember to make mindful decisions and never accept food blindly. There is a difference between being picky about the type of food you eat and being picky about the quality of your food. A foodist sees a clear difference between the two, and if quality standards are met, foodists aim to be as inclusive as possible.

That said, no one is here to judge you for your tastes. If you really can't live without nacho cheese, by all means find a place to fit it into your healthstyle. Quality be damned! At the end of the day only you can decide what value to place on your health and happiness. Just keep in mind that disinclinations toward vegetables or other healthy foods can be overcome if you set your mind to it, and in general quality and value should be your benchmarks for making healthstyle decisions. If health and weight loss are important to you, monitor your weight and adjust your habits until the results start to tip in your favor.

EIGHT

THE WAY YOU MOVE

NEAT, 10,000 Steps,
and Pumping Iron

"If it weren't for the fact that the TV set and the refrigerator are
so far apart, some of us wouldn't get any exercise at all."
—JOEY ADAMS, COMEDIAN

"I really don't think I need buns of steel. I'd be happy
with buns of cinnamon."
—ELLEN DEGENERES

Exercise hasn't gotten much love lately in the world of weight loss.
Most studies have shown that exercising more doesn't lead to a significant drop in body weight, largely because it increases hunger and
people make up for the lost calories with more food. But that doesn't
mean exercise isn't important for your health (some would argue it's
the most important) or even how you look. Although you can certainly hit your ideal weight by tinkering with your diet, adding exercise will make the difference between looking good and looking (and
feeling) amazing. If your healthstyle is important to you, physical
activity is a must.

OH, NEAT!

Fitness doesn't need to start at the gym, so don't worry if you're not the sweating type. In fact, all the little, seemingly extraneous movements you do each day can add up to burn far more calories and have a more positive impact on your overall health than a daily gym trip. The latest research has shown that being sedentary by sitting for long stretches of time throughout the day increases your risk of several chronic diseases, even when formal workouts are part of your schedule.[1] In other words, too much sitting around is not the same as too little exercise—it's much worse. The way to avoid this is to be more active, and not just while you're wearing spandex.

Scientists refer to the activity you do while moving around each day as *nonexercise activity thermogenesis,* or NEAT. Activities that qualify as NEAT include doing dishes, taking a shower, planting a garden, playing with your kids, shoe shopping, chopping vegetables, taking the stairs, punching your little brother, getting the mail, walking to the bathroom, fidgeting, toe tapping, dancing a jig, walking the dog, and even just standing up. NEAT is win-win for busy and lazy people alike, and the more of these small activities you do, the better. Unfortunately, so many jobs require spending long hours in front of the computer* that very few of us come close to our recommended activity level.

Small actions are easy to forget, but this is good news. That it is so easy to add or drop certain activities from your schedule means burning a few extra calories doesn't need to be a chore—in fact, you will hardly notice. All you need to do is build a few simple habits that work some extra movement into your daily routine. Avoid elevators and escalators like the plague, walk to lunch or between floors in your building, do

---

* In case you were wondering, scientists and writers aren't particularly well known for their active lifestyles.

chores more enthusiastically at home, and park farther away in the lot. Just standing up more to get a glass of water or use the restroom* can make a difference. Little activities like these add minuscule amounts of time to your tasks, but contribute significantly to your health.

Unlike structured, high-intensity exercise, walking and other low-intensity movements don't make you hungrier. There's good evidence that increasing your daily activity can burn hundreds of extra calories each day and may be one of the most effective ways to impact your energy balance (i.e., burn more without eating more).[2] Importantly, NEAT correlates with body weight in obese as well as normal-weight individuals, so *everyone* can benefit from extra movement.

Even if you already work out consistently, you should still strive to be less sedentary during the rest of your day. It shouldn't be hard

---

*These tend to go hand in hand.

NEAT Ideas

A few ways to squeeze in the extra mile:

- Take the stairs
- Park farther away
- Get off the train one stop earlier
- Clean house
- Choose activities, not passivities (dancing anyone?)
- Wear a pedometer
- Carry all the groceries at once
- Visit coworkers instead of e-mailing
- Take the long way
- Have walking meetings

to do. I've even found a substantial meditative value in incorporating more physical activity. Several of my most intractable problems have been solved during my long walks with my dog, and I've been plowing through podcasts and audiobooks while running more errands on foot, which I swear makes me smarter.

When you're busy, it's easy to make excuses about why extra effort is impossible or not worth it. But adding more movement to your regular daily activities is far and away the easiest way to lose weight and improve your health, so why not? It's tempting to be lazy and just wait for the elevator with everyone else, even though you know the time it saves you is insignificant. But I hope I've convinced you that it's worth resisting the urge to be sedentary and making an effort to move whenever possible. If you need extra motivation, try making it a game or competing with your friends using social pedometers that are now available.

BE A 10,000-STEP MANIAC

So what is the ideal amount of NEAT? And how do you know if you're getting it? Exactly how noninactive (for lack of a better term) we need to be is a hotly debated topic in the scientific community, but you don't need to sit around and increase your risk of dying while the experts make up their minds. Most people don't get anywhere near the levels of activity that researchers are arguing over, so simply making a concerted effort to move more will make a big difference.

One number that's been thrown around a lot and that works well for most people is 10,000 steps a day. I've found that when I spend the day working at my computer and maybe running a few errands in the car, I clock around 3,000 steps. If you don't move much and don't have a steady gym habit, this is probably close to the number you're getting as well. When I have a fairly sedentary day, but do manage to make it to the gym and squeeze in a little cardio and weight lifting, I'll hit between 6,000 and 7,000 steps. To push myself up past the 10,000-step mark, I need to do something extra, like walk the dog to the park, walk to the gym, or hike to the grocery store (I live in a hilly neighborhood). In my current healthstyle I consistently hit between 10,000 and 12,000 steps per day, and I know that in this range maintaining what I consider my perfect weight is fairly easy. If I walk more than this, I can reliably lose weight. You can see why I've become something of a 10,000-step maniac.

Interestingly, the days when I've hit my highest step counts are almost never gym days. Instead, they tend to be days when I'm running errands on foot downtown (I can easily hit 17,000 to 18,000 steps) or vacation days when I'm exploring a new city. I once walked over 26,000 steps in Tokyo,* and it was one of the best days of my life. Extra movement doesn't need to be painful.

If it isn't feasible for you to spend an additional hour walking your dog each day, there are a few ways to squeeze in extra steps without drastically cutting down on your work time. Standing desks or, better yet, treadmill desks are becoming more and more popular in office settings, particularly as companies try to cut down on healthcare costs and sick days. It's definitely worth asking around the office to see if a new desk is feasible for your workspace—your coworkers might even think you're a genius for coming up with the idea. If a standing desk is impossible, look into getting one of the small pedaling machines that can fit under any standard work desk. Though pedaling isn't the same as walking, it will serve the same function and is far better than nothing, if it's your only option. These only cost around $20.

To make sure you consistently hit your 10,000-step goal, my number one recommendation is to buy and wear a pedometer. Since we know how easy it is to let your NEAT activities slip, tracking

---

* Be sure to wear comfortable shoes if you plan to try this sort of insanity on your own.

your step count will force you to pay attention and keep you honest. It's amazing what a big difference such a small device can have on your healthstyle.*

PUMPING IRON

Obviously I'm a huge proponent of NEAT and 10,000 steps. They work and are enough to change the lives of most people. Yet there are still reasons to consider upping the ante and adding some cardiovascular exercise and strength training to your regimen. As I've mentioned, I make an effort to hit the gym four to six days a week on top of the NEAT activities I've built into my healthstyle. My workouts are precious to me, and I am not a happy camper if I go too many days without training.

Moderate- to high-intensity cardio exercise is one of the best things you can do for your health. It lowers blood pressure, raises your healthy HDL (high-density lipoprotein) cholesterol, improves your metabolism, and generally makes you feel fantastic. Words can't do justice to describe how good it feels to be able to climb the Eiffel Tower without breaking a sweat. Being in great cardiovascular shape, more than any other thing I do, makes me feel as though I'm in control of my body and have the endurance to get through anything. My typical workouts only include about thirty minutes a day on the treadmill, stationary bike, or elliptical machine, but it's enough to make a tremendous impact on my quality of life.

If cardio has the greatest impact on how I feel, strength training gets the trophy for improving how I look. Regardless of how much (or little) it tips the scale, weight lifting can transform the shape of your body for

---

* My favorite device for monitoring activity is definitely the Fitbit pedometer. Small and sleek, it's simple to use and has a long battery life. I clip mine to my undergarments and check my status a few times a day.

the better, and I highly recommend it for both men and women. The same body weight can look very different on a person depending on how muscle is distributed. Don't think of strength training as adding bulk, but as improving shape and adding tone. Women in particular tend to fear the effects of weight lifting, but without testosterone it is difficult for a female to develop large bulging muscles like a male. Instead, strength training creates beautiful lines and curves on a woman's body and helps you look better at every size. I promise, ladies, once you see the changes, you'll never go back. For the dudes, strength training is equally beneficial, though I doubt you fellas need the kind of convincing the girls do. Besides the obvious perks of adding strength and improving physique, weight training also does wonders for your body's resilience and gives you more wiggle room to enjoy your favorite foods.

A final bonus of high-intensity exercises is their impact on energy levels. I was somewhat surprised to learn that vigorous exercise doesn't lower your inclination toward NEAT, but raises it. In one study, scientists measured NEAT three days before and three days after overweight individuals performed either moderate- or high-intensity exercise. There was no measurable change in NEAT until the third day after exercise, when it increased 17 percent after moderate activity and 25 percent after intense activity.[3] That's impressive and shows there could be a synergistic effect of being more active.

I've said that I spend thirty minutes doing cardio exercise whenever I'm at the gym. In addition, my workouts always include a brief (twenty- to thirty-minute) weight-lifting session. My workout partner[*] and I focus on two or three major muscle groups each day and try to get through the entire body (shoulders, chest, biceps, triceps, back, and legs) two times per week. We also do some kind of abdominal or core workout each day. That's it.

---

*A large, muscular male. I only point this out to illustrate that a similar routine can work for many different body types.

10 Tips for Starting and Sticking with Exercise

1. Commit to consistency

This is worth repeating. Make a commitment to sticking with your plan. If you find yourself not able to meet your goals, change them so they're easier.

2. Take baby steps

I jogged around the block for years before I got lost one day, accidentally ran eight miles, and decided marathon training no longer seemed so ridiculous. Don't expect to turn into Superman overnight. For now, just try to stop being Hedonismbot.

3. Pick an exercise that's fun

Not all exercise happens in the gym. Like to climb rocks? Shoot hoops? Swing the bat? Start with the fun stuff and work your way up.

4. Bring a friend, make it competitive

Having a workout partner is one of the most effective ways to be accountable and make your workout fun. Making it a competition is also great for motivation.

5. Join a sports team

Even better than one friend is a group of friends. Intramural sports teams are a fantastic way to squeeze in a few weekly workouts.

6. Get into music, podcasts, and audiobooks

If your schedule isn't conducive to group activities, your iPod has still got your back. Put together an inspiring workout mix, download some of your favorite podcasts and audiobooks, and whistle while you work.

7. Get a dog

You know what takes a lot of energy? Puppies! If you can't get motivated to exercise for yourself, at least do it for Fluffy.

8. Recharge with caffeine

Sometimes a long day can make an evening workout seem impossibly difficult. At times like these, caffeine is your friend. After about half an hour you'll need to work out to burn off that extra energy.

9. Get some nice workout clothes, shoes, and MP3 player

New toys are fun. Sometimes it's the little things that help the most.

10. Reward yourself

Doing something consistently is an accomplishment, even if your actual task seems small and insignificant. If you've been exercising regularly, don't forget to pat yourself on the back for many jobs well done.

If you aren't familiar with the equipment in your gym, find a friend who can show you the ropes or consider hiring a trainer for one or two sessions to show you what to do. Personal trainers these days seem to prefer teaching complicated exercises that involve multiple muscle groups (not to mention strange equipment), so ask them if they can keep it simple for you, so you won't have any trouble doing the exercises on your own. There are certainly benefits from the fancy exercises personal trainers love to teach, but I've found that too often people feel intimidated at the thought of doing these on their own and end up using this as an excuse to not work out as often. If you feel obligated to pay a trainer every time you work out or need to have special equipment to exercise properly, you're creating unnecessary barriers that will likely sabotage your efforts. Good old-fashioned pulls and presses work just as well as the fancy stuff for looking and feeling great.

WHAT IF I DON'T LIKE TO EXERCISE?

You know who you are. As hard as you've tried, you've never liked going to the gym. Maybe you've even hired a personal trainer a few times, hoping the added expense and accountability would be enough motivation to turn you into a regular gym rat. But it didn't work. Every time you've started an ambitious workout program with the goal of getting in shape, something—you're not even sure what—has cut you short before you've reached your goal.

Deep down, though, you know what the problem is: you don't like working out. It's hard, it's uncomfortable, it's sweaty, and the weight room has a weird smell. You don't like the way you look in those stupid clothes, and who even has time for that sorta thing anyway? But still you wonder about those people who are in the gym all the time. What's their secret? How do they stay motivated day after day and year after year? Are they a different species? Or is there something they know that you don't?

Few people on this earth were born with an innate love of the gym. But what generally separates people who like working out from those who don't is simple: fitness. Working out sucks when you aren't in shape. But the good news is that you don't need to become a complete meathead to get to a place where exercise is no longer a pain. Just like learning to cook, once you reach a minimum proficiency level—in this case fitness level—exercise stops feeling bad and starts feeling good. And just like with cooking, the only way to get there is to just do it.*

If you're just starting a workout program, your goal shouldn't be to get buff or lose weight. The first step is getting to a fitness level where you no longer hate to exercise. And for that all you need is consistency. When you first start your program, don't force yourself to do anything too hard or unpleasant; just make sure that you stick with it and never quit. Before I began exercising, I had always hated running. So the first time I went jogging, I told myself I would just run until I got tired. I literally made it about four blocks and went home. After a week or two I was up to eight blocks. That was over ten years ago, and I've since

---

* Dear Nike, please don't sue me.

completed three marathons. Running is no longer my go-to sport, but I'm now the fit person I've always wanted to be.

There's no reason to torture yourself at the gym. Once you're in better shape, you will enjoy pushing yourself a little harder every now and then. But until you get there, just make yourself do something. Anything. Just do it regularly, and don't make excuses.

The key to being consistent is making your workout so convenient/ easy/fun/awesome that not doing it just feels silly.

NINE

RECALIBRATION, TROUBLESHOOTING, AND MAINTENANCE

"Try not. Do. Or do not. There is no try."
—YODA, *STAR WARS*

"Success and failure. We think of them as opposites, but they're really not. They're companions—the hero and the sidekick."
—LAURENCE SHAMES, AMERICAN NOVELIST

"Success is often the result of taking a misstep in the right direction."
—AL BERNSTEIN, AMERICAN SPORTSCASTER

The ideas we've covered so far are enough to free most of us forever from the tyranny of dieting, never again to subject ourselves to long days of lemon juice and cayenne pepper. Naturally though, there are exceptions. If you've spent a decade or more eating a steady diet of processed foods, or if you've gone on and off enough weight-loss programs to make Kirstie Alley blush, you might find that getting back on track is a little tougher than I've made it sound up until this point.

The problem is that what we've been eating for the past fifty years is worse than useless; it actually creates some serious metabolic issues that require special effort to overcome. Insulin resistance is a hallmark of the standard American diet (aptly abbreviated as SAD), and it can make weight loss especially difficult by compromising your normal metabolic responses to food. Though it is usually reversible, insulin resistance requires some special dietary adjustments until normal metabolic function is restored. Other problems like food sensitivities and intolerance can also contribute to stalled weight loss and more subtle health issues. Once you've resolved all your healthstyle hiccups and landed in your happy place, you're ready to enter the final stage of becoming a foodist: lifetime weight maintenance.

METABOLIC MELTDOWN

Make no mistake about it, our Western diet is not normal. The USDA estimates that caloric intake increased 24.5 percent (about 530 calories per person per day) since 1950, with the vast majority of the extra food coming from processed grains (9.5 percent), processed oils (9.0 percent), and added sugar (4.7 percent). Though we're eating more meat than ever, the percentage of fat consumed from meat fell from 33 percent in 1970 to 24 percent in 2000, demonstrating once again that saturated fat isn't the problem.[1]

To put these numbers in perspective, Americans are consuming on average 200 pounds of grain per person per year, up from only 155 pounds in 1950.* This is equivalent to 10 servings per day, even after adjusting for waste and other factors. The USDA also notes that these numbers are an underestimate, since they exclude wheat products not manufactured from flour, such as Shredded Wheat. The sugar situation

---

*This is just an average. I know I hardly eat any processed grains myself, so some of you must be doubling up.

is even worse. Consumption of sucrose (table sugar) and high-fructose corn syrup (HFCS) increased 39 percent from 1950 to 2000.[2] The numbers get more disturbing if you look back two hundred years. According to researchers Stephan Guyenet and Jeremy Landen, who compiled data from the U.S. Department of Commerce and the USDA, the average American consumed only 6.3 pounds of sugar per year in 1822, compared to 107.7 pounds at our peak of sugar consumption in 1999.[3] On his blog Whole Health Source, Guyenet reflects, "Wrap your brain around this: in 1822, we ate the amount of added sugar in one 12-ounce can of soda every five days, while today we eat that much sugar every seven hours." He remarks, somewhat jokingly, that if we follow his sugar consumption graph to its logical conclusion we'll have a diet of pure sugar by the year 2606.[4]

The pre-Victorian era sugar consumption of 6.3 pounds per year would be considered neurotically low by today's standards. In fact, if you announced it as your goal, someone might accuse you of having an eating disorder. It's important to remember, though, that it isn't our ancestors who were abnormal—it's us. Virtually everyone is eating too much sugar. There are exceptions, but if you are not yet making a conscious effort to avoid restaurants and packaged foods, you are almost certainly eating more sugar than you're aware of. Moreover, if you are currently overweight or experiencing metabolic dysfunction, sugar and processed grains are probably the reason.

Our bodies are not designed to be fed this way. As we discussed in chapter 4, there's a happy range in which most of us can consume one type of food in reasonable quantities without much problem. But when you start venturing out of that range (remember the bok choy lady), especially by orders of magnitude as we have with sugars and grains, our bodies lose the ability to deal with foods they could normally handle without issue. These problems manifest as metabolic disorders such as type 2 diabetes and obesity. They also disrupt our normal satiety signals, making us less sensitive to insulin, leptin, and ghrelin, hormones that tell us when we should and shouldn't eat. This is all bad news and ultimately leads to a world of problems known collectively as "diseases of civilization," which include metabolic syndrome, heart disease, hypertension, and cancer.

These problems can be reversed up to a point by eating more vegetables and fewer processed foods, but if you've assaulted your body with flour and sugar for long enough, it can be difficult to get it to return to its normal food responses. In these cases, special steps may be necessary to return your metabolism to a state where it reacts normally to what you put in your body. At the extreme end of the spectrum this could mean using medications to help regulate your metabolic processes, as is the case with type 2 diabetes and prediabetes. But people with any level of metabolic disorder can start to right the ship by eating in a way that resensitizes their body to insulin.

I've mentioned already that there is a place for sweets in a foodist's healthstyle, because life is too short to go without birthday cake for the rest of your life. Some people, however, have trouble tolerating even small indulgences like a single cookie or dinner roll, because their metabolisms have been abused for so long with massive amounts of processed grains and sweeteners. Refined grains and sugars are digested very rapidly, since your body can absorb them almost immediately after they are eaten. When you eat large quantities of these foods (as many people do several times per day), your body experiences rapid blood-sugar spikes. To deal with the influx of glucose, your pancreas secrets insulin to channel the sugar to where it is needed, such as your muscles and brain. The excess sugar—and there's a lot of it—is stored as fat (this also requires insulin).

Think of each cell as having a bunch of little doors* through which blood sugar (fuel) can enter. The doors are normally locked, but when

---

* Insulin receptors, for you biochemistry geeks.

insulin is around, it acts as the key to let sugar in. If there is lots of sugar trying to get into your cells and the cells become too full of glucose, the fuel doors start to disappear and having more insulin around will no longer allow more sugar into the cells. This is insulin resistance, where your body can still produce insulin but is less responsive to it. The excess glucose that cannot enter your cells remains in your blood, a condition known as hyperglycemia. Having too much blood sugar also disrupts liver function, which contributes to body fat accumulation and insulin resistance by a different mechanism. Worse, overtaxing your liver with sugar results in the deposition of fat around your organs, which is the most deadly kind of body fat. Ultimately your pancreas gives out from trying to produce enough insulin to keep up with the glucose overload, and full-blown diabetes develops.

The obvious first step in reversing this cycle is to cut out sugar and processed grains, and this is indeed an effective treatment. Removing refined grains and sweeteners from your healthstyle and replacing them with whole foods lowers the glycemic load of your meals, which is the best-known dietary intervention for improving insulin sensitivity in diabetics.[5] Don't confuse this with the generic "low-carb" diet, which restricts all foods that are rich in carbohydrates and permits unrestrained gorging on any food low in or devoid of carbohydrates.[*] The goal is not to starve yourself of blood glucose, but to stabilize it so that your cells and organs can resensitize to insulin. Becoming insulin sensitive (as opposed to insulin resistant) and getting your metabolism back on track can make a huge difference in how your body responds to changes in your healthstyle. Many people, therefore, may find it worthwhile to spend a brief period of time recalibrating their body for optimal performance.

---

[*] Although I eat fewer processed carbohydrates than most Americans, I certainly don't intentionally restrict my carbohydrate intake for the sake of weight loss. I doubt those who lived in the pre-Victorian era considered themselves low-carb either.

RECALIBRATION

If your body seems resistant to weight loss or you have other health issues you suspect could be diet-related, such as fatigue, digestive upset, or difficulty concentrating, a two- to four-week healthstyle recalibration may help you resolve your problem. Insulin resistance is the most common issue that prevents people from achieving their goals, but other problems such as systemic inflammation or food sensitivities and allergies could also be the cause.

The purpose of a recalibration is to temporarily remove the foods that stimulate these problems until your body is functioning properly. You can then add the foods back slowly and see how you tolerate them. Recalibration is *not* a weight-loss diet, though in the long run it may help you lose weight. Health professionals refer to this as an *elimination diet,* and it is frequently used to resolve diet-related health issues. The recalibration I recommend is not as rigorous as a clinical elimination diet, and obviously you should consult with your physician if you suspect a serious condition. However, this simplified version is a very useful tool for troubleshooting food-related health issues.

A foodist's recalibration requires going at least two full weeks without any of these foods:

- Sugar
- Wheat
- Dairy
- Alcohol

I'll warn you now that the first three days are the hardest and you'll consider punching kittens to get your hands on a chocolate bar. Around the fourth day, though, you'll begin to realize that you may actually survive this ordeal without committing a felony. By day five or six, you should start to feel amazing. Over the next week or so symptoms will resolve, you'll have more energy, your skin will clear up, and your stomach problems will mysteriously disappear. For some people this could take longer,* but two weeks is the minimum time frame in which you're likely to see results.

SUGAR

The reason for cutting out added sugar is obvious. We've already discussed how sugar overload creates insulin resistance, and cutting back on sugar as much as possible is one of the most effective ways to restore insulin sensitivity. Sugar is also unique compared to other foods in that it has addictive properties.[6] People often find it difficult to gradually cut back on sugar and have more success going cold turkey for a few days and then reintroducing it slowly—it's sugar that makes the first few days of recalibration so hard. Once you get through the washout, you'll find it is much easier to keep your sugar consumption under control.

Be careful of hidden sugar sources during recalibration. Desserts are obvious, but most salad dressings and even savory sauces such as ketchup and barbecue sauce are full of added sugars. Check labels and ingredient lists carefully, and always ask at restaurants if you aren't sure. Since one of the goals here is recalibrating your palate to enjoy less sweet foods, you should also avoid artificial sweeteners.

To clarify, I'm not suggesting you eliminate naturally occurring sugars, like the kind in fruit. In fact, fruit is a great weapon for combating the inevitable sugar withdrawal cravings. Instead, we're looking to remove added sugars, specifically sucrose and fructose. Honey is the exception. Even though it's naturally occurring, honey is a concentrated source of fructose and should be avoided during recalibration. It's just two weeks; you'll survive.

---

*Gluten intolerance may require up to eight weeks without wheat for symptoms to resolve completely.

WHEAT

Flour is made from wheat, and whether it's whole grain or not, it'll spike your blood sugar like a Heisman Trophy winner. The other issue with wheat is gluten. Gluten is a protein found in wheat and related grains, such as barley and rye, that can irritate the gut. Wheat allergies and sensitivities are becoming much more common, probably because of the wheat overconsumption trend in the SAD. In extreme cases gluten can induce abnormal immune responses, as is true in celiac disease. There is a wide range in the reactions people can have to wheat and gluten, and some of you may have sensitivities you are not aware of. Unfortunately, laboratory tests for wheat allergies and sensitivities are notoriously unreliable, and the best method for determining wheat and gluten intolerance is still the elimination diet.

If you suspect you have a gluten sensitivity, you may need to be more stringent with your gluten elimination than I recommend here and avoid products that do not naturally contain wheat, but are often contaminated by gluten, such as rolled oats.* You may also need to eliminate gluten for up to eight weeks before symptoms resolve. Consult a physician for assistance in detecting gluten sensitivities. If you don't have any major health concerns, simply eliminating products containing flour for two weeks should be sufficient.

DAIRY

Dairy products are the toughest for me to cut out, particularly because there are several milk-based foods (e.g., yogurt, hard cheese, kefir) that I consider healthy. But dairy creates enough problems for enough people that it's worth a short break to see how you fare.

Dairy gets complicated quickly. Though milk doesn't have a large impact on blood sugar, it shoots insulin off the charts, possibly more

---

* Gluten-free oats that are processed in a clean facility are available in some stores, usually at a premium price.

than white bread.[7] This isn't due exclusively to the lactose (milk sugar), but seems to depend on the whey proteins in milk. It does not appear that the insulin-promoting effect of dairy results in long-term metabolic dysfunction, but since our goal here is to get off the insulin roller coaster, a break is a good idea. The insulin effect of dairy as well as other growth hormones in milk* may also be what mediate the association between milk and acne.[8]

Another issue with dairy is lactose intolerance. I went through years of suffering before realizing that I'm moderately lactose intolerant, and that although a little yogurt here and there is fine, a caffè latte is enough to have me curled on the floor in fetal position for at least an hour. Estimates for the prevalence of lactose intolerance worldwide range from 65 to 75 percent.[9] That's a lot of people. Though rates are substantially lower in Western cultures, lactose intolerance is among the most common food sensitivities, and knowing whether it applies to you is incredibly useful. There are different degrees of lactose intolerance. I can tolerate cheese and fermented dairy products like yogurt. I can even handle a splash of half-and-half in my coffee every now and then, but more than a tablespoon of straight milk or cream, and the stomach cramps come on in full effect. The best way to determine your sensitivity is to stop consuming it for a while and then add it back slowly to see how you react.

ALCOHOL

I love me a glass of nice wine or a well-crafted artisan cocktail. I drink alcohol fairly regularly, and there is a good amount of evidence that it protects against coronary heart disease.[10] Though there have been re-

---

*Some of these hormones occur naturally, while others, such as recombinant bovine somatotropin (rBST), are injected into dairy cows to increase milk production. Use of synthetic hormones is illegal in Canada, Australia, New Zealand, Japan, Israel, and the European Union, but not in the United States.

ports about alcohol increasing cancer incidence, the risks are typically mitigated by a healthy diet that contains plenty of folic acid.[11]

So why do I recommend a two-week break from the sauce? For starters, alcohol lowers your inhibition and makes it much harder to stick to the recalibration. It's hard enough; you don't need any extra excuses. The more important reason, however, is alcohol's effect on your liver. Like fructose (the sugar molecule that is processed by the liver), alcohol promotes body fat accumulation and insulin resistance. For recalibration to be effective, you'll need to be a teetotaler for at least two weeks. Sorry.

WHAT'S LEFT TO EAT?

If the recalibration seems as though it will eliminate 80 percent of your daily calories, fear not. There's plenty left to eat. Remember that cutting out sugar and flour doesn't mean you need to forsake carbohydrates completely. When avoiding refined grains, I rely heavily on beans and lentils to take up a good part of the slack. I also use brown rice, quinoa, and oats to help curb the carb cravings. Of course, you should continue practicing your mindful eating habits, because eating too quickly or too much can still cause substantial blood-sugar and insulin spikes, even if you're eating foods that supposedly have a low glycemic load. But in moderate amounts intact grains and legumes are a fantastic alternative to processed grains. You should also continue to base your healthstyle on a variety of vegetables and fruit as well as sustainable seafood, pastured meats, and poultry. When sugar is what you crave, have a piece of fruit or a glass of mint tea to get you through the hard part. Brushing your teeth works too. The cravings will ultimately pass, so you just need to distract yourself with a healthier option or another behavior (gym time?) to get over the hurdle.

My favorite milk substitute is unsweetened hemp milk. It tastes delicious and has lots of healthy omega-3 fatty acids (ALA) that give it a wonderful creamy consistency. Unsweetened almond and coconut milks are tasty as well. I avoid soy milk, since it is so difficult to find soybeans that have not been genetically modified (GMO). Organic soybeans that are supposed to be non-GMO are often imported from China, and unfortunately there have been enough unsavory practices and food-safety issues in China to make me avoid all Chinese food imports like the plague.* Until the Chinese government develops a track record of cracking down on violations, I'd recommend the same for you. Regardless of which milk substitute you choose, if you choose one at all, remember to check that it doesn't have added sugar (most of them do).

THE MISSING LINK

As important as diet is in improving insulin sensitivity, nothing tops exercise.[12] When you exercise, your muscles rapidly use up the sugar stored in your cells, making room for more. Your muscle cells respond by adding back some of those little doors, so insulin can channel more blood sugar in and it can perform it's natural function: providing you with energy. Exercise restores insulin sensitivity, making it easier for your body to handle the food you eat. If insulin resistance is an issue for you, exercise is essential during recalibration. But don't think you can stop when two weeks are up. Make an effort to build the habit into your daily healthstyle to maintain a strong metabolism. You won't regret it.

Keep in mind that the intensity of your exercise is less important than consistency. Although hard-core exercises like high-intensity interval training (HIIT) are fantastic for improving metabolic markers (particularly if you're short on time, since these exercises can be performed in a fraction of the time a traditional workout takes), consistent

---

*Google "Chinese poison baby formula" for more information.

moderate amounts of exercise are just as effective. Start at the intensity level that is comfortable for you and gradually work to improve your fitness. Strive to add NEAT activities whenever possible as well.

POST-RECALIBRATION

Once two weeks are up, head to the Cheesecake Factory and see if you can eat an entire cheesecake in a single sitting. Just kidding. Don't do that. If your symptoms have mostly resolved after two weeks, you can try slowly adding back foods one at a time and see how you respond. An additional few weeks may be needed to resolve some problems, so feel free to extend your experiment to four or even eight weeks if you feel it may help. Of course, always seek a physician's assistance if you are experiencing serious or chronic health issues.

Pay close attention to how you feel when you're adding back foods, particularly wheat and dairy. Experiment with different amounts until you figure out how much of each kind of food you can handle before it negatively impacts your body, energy, or mood. Try adding back sugar and alcohol as well. Although you can also monitor how you feel when you include these in your healthstyle, they are less likely to have unexpected consequences in small amounts—most of us know what we're getting into when we eat sweets or have a drink. Instead, the goal for sugar and alcohol is to find out how much of these you can include to strike a balance between an amazing quality of life and maintaining your health and weight loss. The precise mix will be a little different for everyone.

WEIGHT-LOSS TROUBLESHOOTING

When troubleshooting weight loss, sugar, flour, and alcohol are the obvious places to show restraint, since they are utterly unnecessary from a nutritional standpoint. With a healthy metabolism, though, you should be able to have them in moderation without much issue. The questions you have to answer for yourself are how often and how much. Some people will experience tremendous success by simply making a few smarter choices in their daily healthstyle. Duhigg and his cookie habit come to mind. Others will require recalibration and may need to be more conservative when choosing indulgences, especially early on. There is never a need to deprive yourself outright or force yourself to settle for less satisfying versions of the foods you love. As we've seen, these tactics can backfire. But budgeting your indulgences for when they're really, truly worth it can substantially benefit your progress if you're still working to improve your metabolism. Don't focus on what you'll be missing; those foods will always be there and you can have them later (remember that trick?). Instead, learn to appreciate the healthier foods you love and make an adventure of discovering new ones.

Recalibration is a way of troubleshooting diet-related health issues and stalled or difficult weight loss. It can be particularly effective if you have more than twenty pounds to lose and suspect insulin resistance is affecting your ability to make progress. By helping restore insulin sensitivity, your body is better able to deal with the food you eat at all your future meals.

For those who don't have any noticeable food issues and have less than twenty pounds to lose, recalibration isn't necessarily the answer. In these cases, focusing on NEAT and mindful eating techniques that improve portion control may be more effective, since just a slight adjustment in your energy balance (calories in versus calories out) likely explains the extra weight. If you're already insulin sensitive (i.e., if you've been following low-carb diets for a while and exercise regularly), adding more slowly digesting carbohydrates such as beans and intact grains can improve your metabolism even further and help you reduce portions of high-calorie foods like meat and cheese. The only way to know for sure is to try different things until you find what works for you.

MAINTENANCE

Maintaining significant weight loss is notoriously difficult, but it is the essence of being a foodist. Building our habits so we can live the awesome life we want is what separates us from the chronic dieters, who suffer through weight-loss programs and endure large swings in body weight. Losing forty pounds in six months and then gaining all but five pounds back by the end of the year is both pointless and demoralizing. But losing thirty-five pounds this year, then another fifteen next year, then another five the following year, and then maintaining that weight into your sixties and beyond, all while eating the best food of your life, is one of the best feelings in the world and is the kind of success foodists strive for. We aren't just losing weight here; we're redefining who we are.

The first essential step is the weight-loss process itself. We've gotten this far by building healthier habits and setting up our environment to optimize our success. As a result, our weight loss occurs slowly, but the decline is steady. Dropping weight rapidly forces our bodies into starvation mode, which slows our metabolism and makes weight maintenance almost impossible. Foodists avoid this fate by building habits that strengthen and improve our metabolism, resensitizing our bodies to insulin through healthy eating and exercise. What we achieve through this is more than just weight loss. Eating like a foodist does something much more powerful: it lowers our bodies' set point.

Set point is a term scientists use to describe the weight at which our body settles naturally and the one it will likely return to if a rapid weight gain or loss occurs.[13] For instance, if your body weight typically fluctuates between 146 and 152 pounds, your set point is likely near 149 pounds (the average). If you go on a strict diet for several weeks and get down to 135 pounds, but then regain the weight over a few months, you will likely return to a weight close to your original 149-pound set point. This works in the opposite direction as well. One weekend of gluttony is unlikely to raise your body weight significantly. So long as your eating binge isn't prolonged, you will probably return to your normal weight within a week or so.

Those who have struggled through bouts of yo-yo dieting know firsthand how difficult it can be to move your set point, but we also know it can be altered. In Western societies people's set points tend to creep upward over time, a recent phenomenon that is likely the result of metabolic disruption caused by our culture's less than ideal food habits and environment. Eating like a foodist undoes this damage, improving your metabolism and helping you reattain your more natural (and likely much lower) set point. When this is the case, it becomes almost as difficult to gain weight as it does to lose it. Lowering your set point, my friends, is the weight-loss holy grail.

As I explained earlier, I was relatively "successful" at dieting and was never considered overweight. My scale fluctuated, but it always hovered about ten to twelve pounds higher than it is today, with swings up to ten pounds in either direction. Today I comfortably rest at my new set point (which is notably five pounds under my original goal weight), and it doesn't take much to keep me within three pounds of this. These may not sound like huge numbers,* but I'm a petite female and I have kept myself in pretty good shape from the get-go. I've had both male and female readers report new set points as low as seventy pounds under their previous weight, and I'm sure even bigger changes are possible for those with more weight to lose.

RESILIENCE

Everyone I've spoken with who has achieved a transformation in their set point describes the feeling with the same word: resilience. "The thing that is most satisfying to me now is knowing that my body has

---

*For my height it meant dropping two sizes.

this resilience," explains the foodist and notoriously fit UCSF neuroscientist Adam Gazzaley, M.D., Ph.D. "In the past if I'd deviate from my diet because of circumstances, which happens, then I'd have to start again from the beginning. A weekend could undo all that progress. And I think for many people at that point they just give up. Now I'm in a more steady state—it feels like homeostasis*—my body does not respond to changes in my diet with such big inflections in weight."

Resilience comes naturally when your set point is established through healthy habits and can be very elusive when it isn't. Shortly after his forty-third birthday, Dr. Gazzaley told me, he decided to approach his diet differently than in the past. After over a decade of struggling with strict low-carb diets and exercise programs, he has now maintained a healthy twenty-five-pound reduction in his set point for over a year. "My thinking was that I've reached the age that I can't keep yo-yoing anymore. As I've gotten older, it's become more and more difficult to lose after bouncing to a high weight every year. The goal was to reach a weight that was sustainable."

Instead of spending a few weeks or months during which he completely eliminates all bread and sugar, foods a pizza-loving native New Yorker has trouble resisting, he lets himself have them when it feels appropriate. "I cut down, but didn't eliminate. I knew that if I entirely eliminated things I knew I really liked that I wouldn't be able to sustain it," Dr. Gazzaley stated. He switched to a foodist's way of eating healthy and working out regularly, but didn't try to push himself to a point that would have derailed him in the past. "I've found a balance of giving myself some leeway when it's really hard not to, then returning to how I ideally eat, which is how I've been able to maintain my weight."

Your body resists dramatic change, which makes it very difficult to move your set point drastically in a short period of time. This is one rea-

---

* Scientists use the term "homeostasis" to describe the tendency of an organism or cell to remain stable internally regardless of changes in the environment.

son traditional dieting fails, and why it is ineffective in the long term to try and skip ahead by losing weight rapidly without establishing the essential habits that keep you there. When you quickly lose a significant percentage of your body weight through deprivation, your metabolism slows—often dramatically. Focusing on healthy habits, however, tends to improve your metabolic markers over time, and weight loss occurs as a result of these changes rather than despite them. When you are a foodist, your body works with you, not against you. "I'm surprised I reached my goal weight as quickly and seamlessly as I did. It didn't feel that bad once I got into a pattern that worked for me, eating in a way that was fulfilling but also helping me lose weight and workout the way I prefer," Dr. Gazzaley told me. "It really wasn't that hard."

For Dr. Gazzaley, monitoring his weight was the key to knowing how often and how far he could push his indulgences while continuing to make progress. He relied on a WiFi digital scale to graph his progression and give himself a quantitative way of measuring the impact of his behaviors. Since he travels often for work, he also purchased a travel scale to help keep himself on track in the situations that he knew to be the most difficult. Monitoring his weight is also how Dr. Gazzaley knows that his set point has moved: "I feel way more stable now than I can remember, so it feels very much like my set point is lower. Even a big violation for a couple of days doesn't change my weight very much."

Having a resilient body means more than not gaining weight back that you've lost. "I've had a couple of weekends that I know in my previous state would have meant a five-pound weight gain that would have been really hard to remove. Now I'll just gain one or two pounds that are gone in a few days. I haven't fluctuated more than three pounds in months," said Dr. Gazzaley. When your body is resilient, it's harder to do the kind of damage that you used to do, and indulgent deviations are easier to correct.

Of course, this doesn't mean it's impossible to move your set point upward again once you've successfully lowered it. When we spoke, Dr.

Gazzaley emphasized repeatedly that he is careful not to take his new set point for granted. Permanent shifts upward or downward, however, require a more prolonged effort than most of us can accomplish in a single weekend.

There are at least two reasons for this stability. First, lowering your set point creates a physical resilience governed by your body's homeostatic mechanisms. You may fidget more or feel an overwhelming urge to go for a run after a big party weekend, or your appetite may be particularly small for the next couple of days. These responses are natural and are your body's way of telling you there's some extra energy to burn—I can hardly wait to get to the gym after an indulgent weekend.

Second, there is a psychological component to a foodist's resilience that stems from the power of habit. Once you've grown accustomed to vegetables and healthy food as the basis of your healthstyle, it becomes very uncomfortable to go for many days without them. I've noticed that if I eat in restaurants for too many meals in a row (it happens to the best of us), I'll start to crave vegetables and salads, which is a cue for me to focus again on my home-cooking habit.

Being hooked on health is a recurring theme for foodists who have successfully altered their set point. Patrick Birke, the man who lost sixty-five pounds after joining a CSA with his family, could only drag himself to the gym to watch episodes of *True Blood* when he first began to change his healthstyle. But after two years, he told me, he now feels an irresistible urge to work out. He currently runs five to ten miles outdoors (no TVs there) a couple of times a week in addition to his regular gym sessions—a healthy habit that is now as hard to break as any unhealthy habit. Dr. Gazzaley describes a similar feeling of "excitement and comfort" when he returns to his food and exercise routine after one of his travel breaks. He looks forward to "getting back in the flow." Habits are resilient actions, and resilient actions lead to a resilient healthstyle.

HOME COURT HABITS

Addicted to salads and workouts? I know it sounds too good to be true, but it isn't magic. Building resilience doesn't come without its struggles, and if you're not vigilant, you can still return to your old habits and undo your success. It is therefore imperative that you identify and maintain the home court habits that are the foundation of your healthstyle.

If you've made it this far, you probably have an excellent idea of which habits are necessary for your continued healthstyle success. Guard these with your life. Your biggest-impact habits are your home court advantage; they are what keep you in the game when life throws you curve balls. My home court habits are eating breakfast, shopping at the farmers market, cooking at home, eating mindfully, walking 10,000 steps a day,* and strength training at the gym. If I'm at home and life is normal, I stick to these without exception, because I know that if they slip, I cannot maintain the rest of my healthstyle without negative consequences. There are always days when the stars don't align and one or more home court habits get missed. Travel, pressing work deadlines, and other special occasions are part of life and sometimes take priority. But if you miss one of your home court habits for too many days in a row, you'll need to make some kind of adjustment to stay in your zone.

Home court habits are the mechanism by which you maintain your weight, just as chores like laundry, dishes, and dusting are the mechanisms by which you maintain your home, flossing and brush-

---

* This is an example of a key healthstyle habit that I was not immediately aware of—remember I inadvertently disrupted it when I stopped commuting to lab. Keep in mind that some of your home court habits may be under your radar and it may take some extra effort to discover them. Monitoring your weight, steps, and food intake are therefore valuable home court habits as well.

ing are how you maintain your teeth, and getting up and going to work every day are the way you maintain your financial stability. Your healthstyle habits are arguably more important than all of these other tasks for your long-term happiness, and they deserve to be treated accordingly. This isn't to say your home court habits should be unpleasant. As we've already discussed, most people enjoy their home court habits and look forward to returning to them. But there are always going to be days when you don't feel like grocery shopping or cooking, and most of the time you should do it anyway. Being lazy is not a special occasion.

If you've built your habits effectively, feeding yourself well shouldn't be difficult, and it is definitely worth it. Though it's easy to mentally compare a pile of sautéed kale with eggs to a super carnitas burrito and assume that the burrito will be faster and more satisfying, this is a mistake. I've done this experiment (several times, in fact), and I can assure you that I almost always overestimate the enjoyment I get from the burrito (especially considering how I feel afterward) and underestimate the deliciousness of the healthier alternative. Cooking at home is also easier, faster, and cheaper than going out, though your mind will falsely try to convince you that it's slower and more work. Kale is always the better choice, and when I've made it, I have never regretted my decision. Don't get me wrong—I love burritos.* I just don't love them as much as I love my health, and saving them for real special occasions helps me appreciate the periodic splurge that much more. So long as you have an arsenal of simple, tasty recipes (your home court recipes) you can throw together with a handful of basic ingredients, defending home court isn't difficult and will continue to get easier as your habits strengthen.

---

*I grew up in Southern California and half my family is Mexican, so good Mexican food is hard to top in my book.

HEALTHSTYLE EVOLUTION

Every time you change jobs, get promoted, commit your life to another person, have a child, move to a new city, alter your travel schedule, or make any of the other big transitions that make life interesting, your habits will have to adapt. Life is full of change, so your healthstyle must evolve to meet its demands. Sometimes the necessary adjustments will be straightforward; sometimes they won't. This might mean something as simple as preparing your lunch at the office rather than at home, but it could also mean revamping your entire workout regimen so you can finish it in half the time.* Your continued success will depend on your ability to experiment and refashion your healthstyle to match your changing circumstances.

The first big shift you'll face is moving from sustained weight loss to weight maintenance. When you've reached your goal weight, you'll be able to splurge a bit more regularly, a phase that requires some trial and error as you find the right balance of fitness and fun that keeps you in your sweet spot. Some people discover that, despite eating treats more often, they continue to lose weight (albeit more slowly) as they attempt to switch from weight loss to maintenance. This is a good sign that your body is settling into its more natural set point, and for most people it is unlikely to be a problem.

There's no reason to let a chart tell you how much you should weigh. Arbitrary scales like the body mass index (BMI) can give you a ballpark number for your ideal weight, but if you're giving your body everything it needs to be healthy, you can determine for yourself where you're the most comfortable, even if it's a little lower or higher than you anticipated. If you feel as though you really are losing too much weight and would prefer not to make up the slack with bread and sugar, eating

---

*Look into HIIT or kettlebells for fast workout options.

more high-calorie healthy foods is your best bet. Dense protein sources such as meat, dairy, eggs, and nuts are a fantastic way to boost your caloric intake without negatively impacting your health. Continue to tweak your healthstyle habits until your weight is stable and your life is awesome.

When you hit a healthstyle snag, your journal and other monitoring tools are your friends. Go back to the basics of measuring and writing down your food, tracking your weight, counting your chews, and using your pedometer, so you can identify the issue. Who knows how long it would have taken me to realize that walking less was what caused me to gain weight after graduation if I hadn't had my pedometer? Problems can't be solved until you know what they are.

As a foodist, you should make it your goal to always focus on real food and build sustainable habits that make smart food choices automatic. Monitoring your actions helps you understand exactly how indulgences affect you, and you can decide from there when they are and aren't worth it. If you accomplish this, you should have plenty of untapped willpower for when your stomach tries to overrule your brain—but of course it shouldn't bother you if your stomach occasionally wins. Your weight is stable, and you know how to stay on course.

PART III

THE DAILY FOODIST

"And remember, no matter where you go, there you are."

—CONFUCIUS

TEN

HOME SAVORY HOME

Your Single Biggest Asset
in Weight Control

"Never work before breakfast; if you have to work before
breakfast, eat your breakfast first."
—JOSH BILLINGS, AMERICAN HUMORIST

"He is the happiest, be he king or peasant, who finds peace in his home."
—JOHANN WOLFGANG VON GOETHE

My health-conscious friends and I unanimously agree that eating out
is the biggest barrier to weight loss. Though it's obvious why eating at
cheap restaurants for every meal isn't going to help you get healthy and
lose weight, excellent restaurants serving real food don't make it that
much easier.

We are fortunate that local, seasonal, high-quality ingredients are
now the standard in almost every big city. We have gastropubs serving
grass-fed beef burgers, street carts offering sustainable fish tacos, and
small neighborhood spots dishing up heirloom vegetables and artisan
ingredients. Basically we're spoiled rotten. There is a downside, though,

to all these wonderful options. Everything tastes amazing and is relatively healthy, so the normal quality over quantity argument doesn't really apply. We have both, so why choose? Even worse, the menus tend to change regularly (often daily) depending on what ingredients are in season, so there's no guarantee that you'll ever be able to enjoy a particular dish more than once. That makes using the "I can eat it later" trick significantly less effective. In other words, the curse of having great restaurants is that it is way too easy to justify overeating.

Home cooking is by far the easiest way I've found to avoid the restaurant trap, and if you tackle it right, it isn't very difficult. We touched on a few of the reasons to take cooking seriously in chapter 6, but I'm sure there are still some of you with reservations.* Chapter 10 will walk you through the basics. Take your time and build your skills at a pace you're comfortable with, and don't let the occasional kitchen mishap keep you from trying again. Start with the easy meals like breakfast and lunch and work your way up from there. It will become fun and easy for you eventually, but the only way to get there is to keep at it.

BREAKFAST OF CHAMPIONS

Breakfast is your slam dunk meal. It's fast, it's simple, and healthy choices are usually delicious. Affordable breakfast supplies are available almost anywhere, and special equipment isn't necessary. Most important, if you make a healthy breakfast one of your home court habits, you virtually guarantee that 30 percent of your daily meals are healthy and contributing positively to your healthstyle. Since automatic health is what we're after, breakfast is a foodist's best friend.

An ideal breakfast has a low glycemic load and contains a good amount of protein. Not only does this encourage your body to use your breakfast calories as fuel rather than storing them as fat; it also

---

* Literally.

improves your metabolic response to subsequent meals throughout the day.[1] This means that one consequence of eating a healthy breakfast is that, no matter what you choose for lunch (and possibly dinner), your body will handle it a little better than it would have if you ate something made of processed grains and sugars or skipped breakfast altogether. That's pretty powerful. Of course, this doesn't mean that you should use breakfast as an excuse to eat an unhealthy lunch. You should generally use your home court advantage to try to eat as healthy as possible when in your regular routine. But small, positive impacts do add up and over the long run work to sensitize your body to insulin and improve metabolism.

Just as important, healthy habits beget more healthy habits. Starting the day with a positive healthy action might inspire you to pack a healthier lunch or cut back on the sugar in your coffee. These may feel like small acts, but they can have a huge psychological impact on your ability to make progress and could ultimately influence what you buy later at the grocery store or help you choose the gym over lying on the couch with a bag of chips. Never underestimate the power of baby steps.

As long as you're eating real, whole foods and not processed junk, what exactly you choose for breakfast doesn't matter much. I recommend finding a few simple breakfast options you enjoy that you can put together while you're practically asleep. My personal breakfast choices tend to cycle every year or so. Currently I'm in the habit of making my own muesli (see recipe, p. 103), which I add a little water to and then microwave for two minutes. It cooks up just like oatmeal; only it's tastier because it is filled with nuts, seeds, and raisins. I top it with a generous heap of cinnamon and a splash of unsweetened hemp milk. It's delicious and keeps me satisfied for hours. In the past I used to sprinkle a smaller amount of dry muesli onto a serving of plain yogurt. Once you stir it around, the muesli softens, and the mix is really tasty. It's good with cinnamon or fruit as well.

8 Reasons Regular Guys Should Learn to Cook

Some guys I know don't consider cooking a worthwhile venture. Other than the occasional stint behind the grill, they'd rather bask in blissful ignorance than feed themselves in more than three steps: stab, chew, swallow.

But ask any woman (or man who already knows how) why it is better to be a kitchen-savvy dude and you'll start to see what these guys are missing. Whether it's because they think it takes too much time or too much effort or wrongly assume it's a woman's job, men who never learn to cook are losing a huge opportunity to take their man skills to the next level.

1. Chicks dig it

There isn't a woman alive immune to a man who can make her a delicious meal. Step up to the plate boys, we're begging you.

2. Life skills are manly

You can fix your car, hunt wild animals, and build a campfire. Shouldn't you know how to feed yourself without a drive-thru?

3. You'll save money

Although there's a good chance you're single if you never learned to cook (see point #1), a home-cooked meal is a much cheaper date night (or singles night) than dinner for two at Chez Fancy—particularly with the 150 percent wine markup common at most restaurants.

4. It's faster than going out

Fancy date meals aside, cooking at home is almost always faster than going out—as long as you know what you're doing. Once you have a few basic skills down, you can stop wasting your time in fast-food spots simply because you don't know what else to eat.

5. Guy Fieri shouldn't be better than you at anything

Food Network star Guy Fieri has bad hair, bad clothes, and ridiculous sunglasses, but the dude knows how to cook. Are you going to let him upstage you like that? Of course you aren't.

6. Your puppy (aka girl magnet) will eat better

My notorious, adorable puppy, Toaster,* loves salad scraps (sugar snap peas are his favorite), eggs, meats, fish, and pretty much anything else we're willing to share. A balanced diet is as good for dogs as it is for people (just don't give them onions, garlic, or grapes).

7. You might lose weight

Cooking is one of the easiest ways to improve your diet and stick to reasonable portions. This is a recipe for weight loss, if you're willing to swallow it.

8. You might like it

Cooking is relaxing, fun, creative, and purposeful. It can also result in delicious eats. Why wouldn't you want to add it to your tool belt?

---

* Toaster was named San Francisco's Cutest Dog in 2011. He has a trophy and everything.

Scrambling, frying, or boiling eggs is another easy, tasty, and satisfying breakfast. I typically pair them with something spicy, like salsa or kimchi, and something green, like sautéed kale. Try sprinkling a little smoked paprika on a fried egg for an absolutely mind-blowing breakfast experience. If I don't have any greens, I'll sometimes start with some beans or lentils, add a few chopped herbs and vegetables (think carrots, cucumber, tomato, etc.), splash on a little oil and vinegar, place a fried egg right on top of the pile, and dig in. Yum. Whatever you choose to have for breakfast, just make sure you enjoy it, because habits don't form without a reward.

8 Reasons Awesome Girls Should Learn to Cook

I know a few girls who enjoy cooking, and even more who like to bake. But there is also a group who can't even boast the grill skills my regular guys have in spades. I know these girls well, because I used to be one.

When I was in college, saying I was a "bad cook" would have been generous. I couldn't cook anything—I even burned water on occasion and was generally afraid of stoves, pans, and ovens. I couldn't prepare any food that required more than a can opener and microwave, and fixing these flaws was not high on my priority list.

I only changed my tune when I got to graduate school, learned how amazing food could taste when great ingredients are prepared properly, and realized I could no longer afford to eat out in all the fabulous restaurants on my student salary. Unwilling to sacrifice the quality of food I was eating, I forced myself to start shopping at the farmers market and preparing my own meals. This switch changed my life for the better, and I would never go back to my kitchen-free days.

But why was I such a brat about it in the first place? Honestly, I thought I was above cooking. I was busy building my career and had better things to do than slave away in the kitchen, thankyouverymuch. Cooking was for stay-at-home moms, I thought, not for ambitious girls like me. Who has time to be so domestic? I was a jackass and have since learned the error of my ways. This one is for all you awesome girls out there who still don't know the value of being kitchen savvy.

1. It's still hot

I'm sure you have no trouble attracting men with your intellect, but no matter how smart and beautiful you are, guys always melt for a girl who can cook an amazing meal. You may have already gotten into college, but extracurriculars still matter.

2. Cooking makes you beautiful

Nothing is more attractive than a woman who radiates health. Cooking nutritious food at home will give you sparkling eyes, shiny hair, healthy nails, and glowing skin.

3. Good food makes you smarter

Junk food creates spikes and dips in blood sugar that make you tired and kill your ability to concentrate. Cooking healthier food at home will give you the focus to stay sharp all day.

4. Cooking is more efficient

Going out may seem quicker because there is no prep or cleanup, but in the long run it actually takes more of your time. Once you have it down, you can make yourself a solo meal and have your kitchen back in working order in about thirty minutes. Win.

5. You'll save money

Being a girl is expensive. And if you're the type who likes to splurge on designer brands, every dollar counts. Cooking at home is a great way to save money on food, freeing it up for you to use on other things.

6. It keeps you slim

For most people I know, eating out is the single biggest factor in their ability to control their weight. At home you have complete power over everything you eat, and when you cook healthy foods, this works to your advantage.

7. You might one day be a mom

You may have your eye on the prize today, but if you ever plan to raise a family, your life will be a lot easier if you pick up some kitchen skills beforehand. Processed foods are bad for you and even worse for kids. Plan ahead for your future healthy family.

8. You might love it

Cooking is like art and science all rolled into one. It allows you to build skills, be creative, and de-stress, and when you're finished, you have a wonderful and delicious product to enjoy (and show off on Instagram). Cooking is more mentally stimulating than I ever imagined, and it is worth exploring for its own sake.

WHAT IF I'M NOT HUNGRY IN THE MORNING?

If you aren't in the habit of eating first thing in the morning, it can sometimes be difficult to start. Many people complain that they are not hungry in the morning and forcing themselves to eat makes them nauseated. There could be a few reasons for this. Dehydration is a common reason people do not feel hungry in the morning. Get in the habit of drinking plenty of water, particularly before bed and in the morning. Another reason you may not be hungry in the morning is that you've eaten too large a dinner or eaten too late at night. These things can also be associated with insomnia, so if you are having trouble sleeping, eating a lighter, earlier dinner might be helpful. Make an effort to build consistent eating habits, so that all your meals occur at roughly the same time each day. If you get to the point where you wake up hungry in the morning, you know you are making progress.

COFFEE AND TEA

It's hard to mention breakfast without also mentioning everyone's favorite morning vice: caffeine. We love it, so it's got to be bad for us, right? Actually, it's fine. If we're talking about real coffee and tea—not the blended sugar bombs that cost $4 at your local coffee chain—then the science is pretty convincing that both tea and coffee do more good than harm.

Coffee is in fact a rich source of polyphenols and antioxidants and has long been known to protect against liver disease.[2] It also appears to protect against several kinds of cancer, including cancers of the liver, uterus, and potentially the colon.[3] Coffee also improves insulin sensitivity, and type 2 diabetes is less common in both people who drink regular coffee and those who drink decaf.[4] Caffeine and coffee enhance cognitive performance as well and appear to protect against Alzheimer's disease,[5] Parkinson's disease,[6] and other forms of dementia and cognitive decline.[7] For you jocks, it also helps with athletic performance.[8] The greatest concern about coffee and caffeine for many years centered on individuals with high blood pressure. However, recent reviews of the data indicate that, although caffeine does temporarily raise blood pressure for about three hours after consumption, there is no long-term increase in risk of hypertension from drinking coffee.[9] In fact, at high levels (four cups per day or more) coffee seems to have a protective effect,[10] possibly from the polyphenols or other antioxidants. Impressive, right?

There are still downsides to coffee, but they are pretty tame compared to those of some of the other horrors we eat. Because coffee has a mild diuretic effect, some have suggested it can be dehydrating. However, this hypothesis is not supported by the data, and coffee drinkers ultimately get a net increase in fluids from drinking their morning brew.[11] The biggest issue with coffee is how it can affect your quality of sleep. If you have difficulty falling or staying asleep, cutting back on coffee or limiting the hours you consume it to earlier in the day could probably help.

Another serious reason to be careful with coffee is the addictive element. Although great coffee is one of nature's most wonderful gifts to humankind, there is a huge difference between enjoying coffee and needing coffee. At several points in my life I've fallen in the latter category, and I can attest that the headaches and mood swings that appear when you don't get your morning fix are very unpleasant. After I defended my thesis I made an effort to switch from coffee to tea, and I'm happy I did. My goal wasn't to ditch caffeine completely, just to moderate the dose, so that if I'm on vacation I don't need to inject myself with espresso to get out of bed. Tea has been a wonderful substitution, and its spectrum of flavors is far more nuanced than I ever imagined. The health benefits of tea are equal to if not better than those of coffee, and I still get to enjoy the occasional cup of joe.

BATCH COOKING

Once you get past breakfast, cooking at home requires a bit more thinking. Oftentimes what holds us back from entering the kitchen is not knowing what the base of our meal is going to be. Even if you have a decent supply of tasty, fresh vegetables in the house, you need something with a bit more protein to make it feel like a real meal. But figuring out what this should be can be daunting, since protein-rich foods like meat and legumes can take a while to prepare.

Enter batch cooking. The best way to avoid having to start a big meal from scratch every time you want to eat is to cook a lot of something at once and save it for later. It wouldn't be impossible, but it would certainly be more challenging for me to cook at home as often as I do if I didn't prepare foods ahead of time. Beans, lentils, and grains lend themselves particularly well to batch cooking; it takes only a small amount of additional planning to prepare them in large batches that can be used as a base or supplement for meals throughout the week. If you're extra clever, you can even freeze some and have them on hand at any time. A scoop or two of beans, lentils, or grains make an excellent base for a salad or can be thrown into a vegetable stir-fry to make it more substantial. They add texture and flavor to salads and soups and can be mixed with almost any other ingredients you have on hand to make a meal more filling.

BEANS, BEANS, THE MUSICAL FRUIT

Beans get a bad rap. No matter how enthusiastically I tell people that beans and lentils are a game changer for weight loss, I inevitably get a sideways glance followed by an overly polite question about the potential for unpleasant digestive issues. No, beans don't make you fart. At least they don't have to, if you prepare them right. The gas-producing quality of beans comes from your body's inability to digest some of

Super Simple Beans

Place a few cups of dried beans in a bowl and cover with water. Let them soak for several hours on the kitchen counter. Cover them with a plate if you're worried about dust or bugs or put them in the fridge if you live in a warm climate. The skins will crinkle for the first few hours of soaking; add more soaking water if it looks as though they need it. When the skins are smooth again and the beans have plumped up, they're ready to be cooked. Be sure to pour off the soaking water and rinse the beans thoroughly.

There's no wrong way to cook beans. Personally, I prefer to cook them in a simple beef stock. Vegetable stock works nicely too if beef stock isn't your thing, and even water will suffice. (You may need to add a little salt when the beans are done cooking if you use water instead of stock.) Beans absorb flavors and seasonings easily, so adding onions, peppers, garlic, celery, carrots, bay leaves, and other spices is wonderful, but your beans will then have those flavors for all the dishes you use them in. I keep the flavors simple during the initial cooking and then add spices later to match the mood of the dish I'm making.

Since I like my time in the kitchen to be as efficient as possible, I always cook my beans in a pressure cooker, which shortens the cooking time substantially. If you aren't in a hurry, feel free to simmer them for 1 hour or so on the stovetop instead. They're done when they're tender, but not falling apart. Follow the instructions on your pressure cooker for optimal cook times, but in my experience soaked beans take about 10 minutes under pressure.

the carbohydrates in beans called oligosaccharides. When these oligosaccharides reach your lower intestine, bacteria break them down, producing gas.

Fortunately, removing these oligosaccharides is easy, because they are water-soluble. If you start with dry beans, an overnight soak will wash out all the offensive sugars and sap the music-producing qualities of these lovely legumes. Soaking also helps beans cook faster and makes their nutrients more digestible. After soaking your beans, discard the soaking water and use fresh water for cooking to prevent digestive issues. Similarly, if you use canned beans, thoroughly rinse off the canning liquid, which contains most of the gas-producing oligosaccharides.

I strongly recommend cooking with dried beans rather than canned, since their flavor and texture are light-years better. You'll also find a more interesting variety of dried beans,* which makes your cooking adventures a lot more fun. There's nothing wrong with canned beans per se, and if you're in a time crunch, they can really come in handy. But your food should be delicious and life should be awesome, and spending a little more effort to make yourself food you're actually excited to eat is more than worth it.

Cooking beans tends to take a similar amount of time no matter how many you make, so cooking big batches and using them throughout the week is a fantastic way to save time. Beans can be used at breakfast, lunch, and dinner to add substance, flavor, and texture to almost any ingredients you have in the house.

---

*I adore the heirloom beans from Rancho Gordo and Zürsun Farms.

5-Minute Lunch

The Tastiest, Healthiest Bean Salad on the Planet

Don't worry, this is not one of those nasty three-bean salads your well-meaning aunt brings to picnics. Beans are one of the absolute best go-to foods when you want something tasty and satisfying. Feel free to substitute any vegetables you have or like better for the ones in the recipe or use lentils instead of beans. This dish turns out differently every time I make it, depending on what I have in the house, my mood, and of course the season. In the summer, for example, I tend to use cucumber, French radish, and a handful of arugula. Also feel free to experiment with different oils, vinegars, citrus, herbs, salts, and spices (smoked paprika is a great addition). I use this dish most often for a light lunch or substantial snack. It can be served warm or cold or can be made into a full meal by adding a fried egg (or other protein) on top with a side of greens. These instructions are for a single serving, but it scales easily.

Heirloom Bean Salad with Winter Vegetables
SERVES 1

1 cup cooked Rancho Gordo pinquito beans
2 small or 1 medium carrot, thinly sliced
¼ cup sliced lo bok or daikon
½ green onion, finely chopped
2 tablespoons fresh parsley, chopped
1 tablespoon olive oil or nut oil
1 teaspoon rice or red wine vinegar
Salt and pepper

Place the beans in a bowl and add sliced vegetables, green onion, and parsley. I tend to go heavy on the herbs, because they add such a wonderful freshness, but feel free to experiment with the amount you like.

You're welcome to mix the vinaigrette beforehand, but if you're lazy like me, you can just add oil and vinegar directly to the bowl along with some salt and pepper and any other spices you choose. Gently stir the mixture with a spoon, taking care not to damage the beans. Adjust salt and pepper and enjoy.

LENTILS

Lentils are the lazy person's bean. Because they are much smaller, lentils cook up in a fraction of the time of beans and without the burden of a pressure cooker. Although all lentils are wonderful, I prefer the varietals that keep their shape after cooking rather than turning into a mushy soup. This enables me to be imprecise with my cooking method (I just boil them in some salted water until they're tender) and use them in a wider variety of dishes. My favorite lentils to cook with are French green lentils (*lentilles du Puy*) or black beluga lentils. In my experience they cook the fastest and have the best flavor.

Like beans, lentils can be used to bolster any dish. But unlike beans, you can decide to make them at the last minute. In twenty to thirty minutes you can have a delicious, steaming pile of fresh lentils that store wonderfully in the fridge for several days. Always keep a hefty supply of lentils in your pantry, and you'll always be able to make a meal.

GRAINS

Rice, quinoa, farro, and other grains are another group of foods that make more sense to cook in large batches, because it's just as easy to cook three cups as it is to cook one. I cook all grains the same way: boil until done. Rice is the only exception; with it I do an additional steam step to give it that characteristic sticky/fluffy consistency.

A huge perk of cooking large batches of grains is that they freeze beautifully and can be stored in individual serving sizes. I always have a handful of rice balls in my freezer that can be used for anything on a moment's notice. To freeze your grains, first cool the pot briefly in the refrigerator or submerge the bottom of the pot in cold water, so that you don't have plastic coming into contact with hot food.*

Tear off squares of plastic wrap (same length as width) and scoop individual rice servings (about a half cup) into the middle. Fold the plastic over the rice like a square taco and press down on the rice and compress the ball to remove air and pack the stray grains into the ball. Fold the excess plastic (top of the taco) back over the rice, then bring

---

* Plastics have chemicals that can leach into foods when heated, so never add anything warm to plastic and always transfer food to ceramic or glass before microwaving.

How to Prevent Gas and Other Digestive Problems Caused by Healthy Eating

The number of questions I get from people about bloating, gas, and other digestive problems is not small, and since it is a sensitive subject, I'm sure the questions I get represent just a fraction of the concerns out there.

It's not uncommon to experience digestive discomfort when you change your diet. For one thing, any drastic change in eating can be a shock to your system, even if it's for the better. Also vegetables, legumes, and other healthy foods contain a number of nutrients such as oligosaccharides, soluble fiber, and natural sugars like fructose that can produce excess gas in the intestine.

Fortunately, several remedies can help prevent the embarrassment and discomfort caused by eating these foods. However, it is important to remember that everyone's digestive environment is unique, and different things will work for different people. This means you'll need to experiment with the following tactics in order to identify what works best for you.

1. Chew thoroughly

When food reaches your intestine that has been only partially digested, the bacteria in your gut cause the food to ferment, producing a substantial amount of (smelly) gas. More chewing helps your stomach acids do their job more effectively and can dramatically reduce the bacterial gas that gets formed.

Chewing is even more important when you're eating vegetables and high-fiber foods, because they are more difficult to break down in your mouth and stomach than, say, a slice of white bread. This means you need to grow accustomed to chewing each bite of food more than you did for processed foods.

2. Take smaller bites

For the same reason it is important to chew, taking smaller bites can help ensure that large chunks of food do not reach your intestine undigested. People who take smaller bites also tend to eat slowly, which helps prevent overeating—another cause of poor digestion.

3. Don't get too full

Overloading your stomach will eventually overload your gut, which can prevent proper digestion and cause discomfort. Both chewing and taking smaller bites can help with this, but you can also use our tricks to eat less without noticing (p. 41) if this is a problem for you.

4. Eat balanced meals

On a similar note, you don't want to overload your gut with one kind of food. If all you're eating is a giant mound of vegetables for dinner and you're having trouble digesting it, try balancing out your meal with more protein, starch, and fat. These will enable you to feel satisfied with a smaller volume of food (remember point #3) as well as decrease the load of any one nutrient that may be causing problems.

5. Increase vegetable and fiber intake gradually

Going from fast food every day to lots of vegetables can be shocking to your system. The bacterial environment in your gut is accustomed to a certain flow of nutrients, and drastically changing this can cause gas and bloating. Your gut can acclimate to a new diet over time, and the key to avoiding discomfort is to make changes gradually. If you're really struggling with all that broccoli, cut back a little and see if it helps. Once you're comfortable, you can try adding more if you like.

6. Experiment with probiotics

Most of the gas in your intestine is produced by bacteria, but there are also strains of bacteria that have the opposite effect. Adding probiotic foods to your diet can help populate your gut with helpful bacteria that can ease digestion and reduce gas. There are several strains of probiotic bacteria, and research suggests that different strains work better for different people. Experiment with different kinds, and when you find one that works, stick with it to maintain the benefits.

Examples of probiotic foods are yogurt, sauerkraut, kimchi, kombucha, and miso. Keep in mind that when you cook these foods, you will kill some of the active bacteria, so try to eat them raw whenever possible.

7. Soak your beans

Beans are infamous for producing excess intestinal gas, but proper preparation can mitigate this problem. Instead of buying canned beans, get dry beans and soak them for at least six hours before cooking them. Soaking beans and discarding the soaking water eliminates the majority of the oligosaccharides that cannot be digested, reducing bacterial fermentation and intestinal gas. If you do buy canned beans, rinse them thoroughly, since most of the oligo-saccharides are in the canning liquid.

8. Eliminate wheat

Some people have chronic stomach problems that are caused by food intolerance. Wheat sensitivities are the most common, and eliminating wheat and gluten is often the only solution. If you've tried everything and are still in pain, it may be worth giving up wheat and gluten for four to eight weeks to see if it helps. If it works, now you know. If it doesn't, at least you tried.

9. Eliminate dairy

Like gluten, many people have sensitivities to lactose, the sugar in milk, that can develop over time. Cutting it out for a few weeks is an easy way to tell if it is a problem for you.

10. Avoid fake sugars

Sugar alcohols such as sorbitol and xylitol can cause digestive problems similar to the oligosaccharides found in beans. If you've been relying on artificial sweeteners to cut back on real sugar, this may be a cause of your digestive issues.

11. Reduce fresh and dried fruit intake

Fructose can ferment in the gut, and too much will result in gas and discomfort. If you've drastically increased your fruit intake, this may be problematic for your digestion. Cut back until you find the amount you can tolerate.

(*Note:* I'm giving you the benefit of the doubt and assuming you've eliminated most of the high-fructose corn syrup from your diet already.)

12. Use medication

Beano is an enzyme formulation that helps with digestion of oligo-saccharides that can cause gas. If you simply cannot miss out on your grandpa's famous chili, popping the occasional Beano at the beginning of your meal should help.

On the other hand, if you still haven't figured out what you're sensitive to and find yourself in an unpleasant state, Gas-X is an effective form of relief that can be used on occasion. It takes twenty to thirty minutes to work. As always, be sure to follow the safety instructions when taking any medication.

each end to the center, and tie a half knot so the rice looks a bit like a ball. Put all the rice balls into a freezer bag and store in the freezer. Those little plastic fold-top sandwich bags work great for this too. Shake the rice down into one corner, grab it with your hand and squeeze the air out, twist the top, and lay the pouch on the counter with the twist underneath it. Pack into a freezer bag the same way, twist underneath, and when it's frozen, it won't matter that the top is not tied.

To thaw, remove a rice ball from the freezer and allow it to sit on the counter for a few minutes until you can untie the knot without leaving little pieces of plastic stuck in the folds of rice. If you forget to do this (as I always do), you can run the knotted plastic under tepid water until you can untie it. Place the unwrapped frozen rice ball in a small bowl and microwave on high for one or two minutes.

Alternative grains like quinoa or my favorite, farro, are even easier than rice and can be similarly stored. Quinoa cooks up in just ten to fifteen minutes, depending on the varietal. Just rinse the grains and then boil in excess water until tender. Farro takes a bit longer, about twenty to thirty minutes depending on how much you make, but the protocol is the same.

How to Cook Perfect Rice Without a Rice Cooker

This recipe works for any style of rice. I prefer short-grain brown rice for most dishes, but sometimes cook long-grain basmati rice or the delicious and nutritious Japanese haiga white rice.

Place 2 to 3 cups of dry rice grains in a large saucepan. Add cold water until it is almost full, and use your hand to swirl the rice around and loosen any dirt and dust. When the rice settles back to the bottom, dump the water off the top and repeat. Continue to rinse the rice until the water is almost perfectly clear, about four or five times.

After the last rinse, add cold water to the rice until you have at least three times the volume of water as rice. Don't worry too much about the amount and err on the side of excess. This is especially important with brown rice, which absorbs more water than white rice.

Place the rice and water on the stove and turn the heat on high. When the rice begins to boil, reduce heat to medium and continue to simmer, uncovered. This is a good time to start the rest of your dinner.

Check on the rice grains after about 15 minutes by grabbing a few out with a fork and testing them for tenderness (squish between your fingernails or teeth). Rice becomes opaque when it cooks, so there is no point in checking it while it is still somewhat translucent.

Once the rice does start to turn opaque, check tenderness every 2 to 5 minutes. If too much water evaporates and the rice starts to look soupy, add more water. You should add enough water at the beginning to avoid this.

Simmer the rice until it is *almost* tender enough to eat. If you aren't sure when it is ready, imagine you are an impatient person who wants the rice to be finished as quickly as possible, so you decide the rice is done and serve it, but later regret that decision because the rice is ever so slightly *al dente*. If you think it's ready (this is not an exact science, so don't overthink it), dump off all the liquid. A mesh strainer or splatter guard works nicely for this (simply hold it tightly over the pot and dump the water into the sink). Place the pot with rice back on the burner and reduce the heat to as low as it will go. Cover the rice and set a kitchen timer for 5 minutes.

After 5 minutes turn off the burner and set the timer for another 5 minutes. Do not lift the lid during this process unless you are concerned that you cooked the rice too long and want to check if it is getting too sticky.

After the rice has sat for 5 minutes, remove the lid, fluff the rice with a fork, and serve. If for some reason you think you overcooked the rice, you can skip the steaming step and just let the drained rice sit covered with the burner off for 5 minutes. If you undershoot, you can always extend the length of the steaming step.

LUNCH

If you work from home, lunch should be as much of a slam dunk as breakfast. A simple, fast, and delicious lunch doesn't require any real cooking skills. If you've got batches of beans, lentils, or grains in the house, all you need is a few fresh vegetables, some herbs, and a simple vinaigrette and you've got a great meal. Legumes or grains can be the basis of a warm or cold salad, or you can add them to a regular green salad for more texture and density. Keep in mind that even if you don't work at home, any of these ideas can be packed up and taken to the office.

Lunch is a perfect meal to experiment with if you're new to cooking, since it is less elaborate than a typical dinner. Play around with different vegetables and test new flavors like ginger or curry in salads or simple stir-fries. Try cooking eggs* in new ways and add different spices. As long as you do your best to include some kind of vegetable and minimize your processed grains and sugars, you're golden.

---

*Eggs are one of my favorite go-to lunches, since they're so fast, healthy, and delicious.

Lunch is also a fantastic way to dispense with leftovers. Obviously you can eat any extra food you have the way it is, but it's also fun to turn it into an entirely new creation. Meats are a fantastic ingredient to play with and make a great addition to salads, stir-fries, soups, or egg dishes. Leftover vegetables can be added to beans or grains with a dash of olive oil, salt, and pepper (and maybe a little vinegar if it tastes flat). Toss in some fresh greens or herbs to brighten your meal with color and flavor. Imagination is your only limit.

DINNER

In my experience, dinner is when the home-cooking anxiety usually sets in. Whether you're cooking for yourself or a whole family, at least a little bit of foresight and planning are required to make dinner a smooth ride. But fear not; it isn't as hard as it sounds.

Start with the Foodist Plate we discussed in chapter 4 (and printed again on p. 230). Half your plate should be vegetables, and the more different kinds you can throw in, the better. It's a good idea to have something green in there on most nights. The other half of your plate is more nebulous. You can have a perfectly healthy dinner that completely neglects either the meat or bean component, but including both will probably be the most satisfying. Depending on my mood, the ingredients I have at home, and the cuisine I feel like making, dinner can look wildly different on any given night and still fit the model. One night might be Japanese-style baked fish with rice and bok choy, and the next might be marinated flank steak with Cuban-style beans and grilled veggies. The options are endless, and this is a blessing.

It can often help to have a rough meal plan at the beginning of the week, so you have an idea of what to pick up while you're shopping. Though it's common practice to choose some recipes and then go shopping for ingredients (and this is a reasonable place to start if you're very new to cooking), I tend to use the opposite approach. You can never be 100 percent certain of what you're going to find at the farmers market each week, so having a long list of must-have ingredients for your recipes is likely to be frustrating. A shopping list with items you can't get will leave you scrambling, running around the market looking for absent ingredients or inferior substitutes. No fun. The last thing you want to do is turn the farmers market into a source of anxiety. Besides, one of the best things about shopping at the farmers market is discovering new and interesting foods. It takes an open mind and curious eyes if you hope to discover your next favorite vegetable (trust me, it's out there), and a rigid shopping list will only hinder your exploration. That said, you don't want to end up with a pile of random vegetables and no obvious meals.

The best meal-planning strategy combines both structure and flexibility. Start with an idea of what you want to accomplish, and then let the season's offerings nourish your spirit of adventure and round out your menus. The first thing to consider is how many meals you want

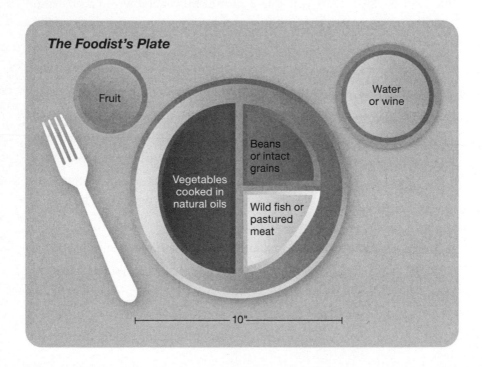

The Foodist's Plate

Fruit

Water or wine

Vegetables cooked in natural oils

Beans or intact grains

Wild fish or pastured meat

10"

to get from your purchases (e.g., four dinners, three lunches) and what their main courses might be, given that a few will probably repeat, since you're so skilled in batch cooking. It's perfectly okay to have one or two things in mind you know you want to make and let the rest of your meals be inspired by wandering through the aisles and seeing what catches your eye.

As you discover which foods will be the focal points of your meals, start to think about how you might like them cooked (even if you don't know how to cook them that way yet; Google can help with this later). Think about what other flavors usually taste good with what you're buying—consider herbs (parsley, thyme, mint, cilantro, etc.), proteins (meats, fish, eggs, legumes), and side dishes. If you can't think of anything, try to remember how these foods have been served to you in a restaurant. If you still aren't sure what other flavors would be a good choice, ask the vendor you are buying from. Farmers are usually pretty good at cooking the foods they grow. Keep in mind that most seasonal foods are delicious cooked in a little olive oil and garlic with a sprinkle of salt. So don't feel you have to get super fancy to make something delicious.

Out of all the different ideas you had for meals, choose the ones that can be made with common flavors and overlapping ingredients. See what is available and purchase the ingredients that are the most versatile. Flavors that can be included in several different dishes give you the flexibility to change up your meal plans in the middle of the week, if you are suddenly struck with inspiration. As your ideas solidify, be sure to collect all the elements you need. iPhone apps can be particularly helpful with this if you want to double-check ingredient lists for things you may have forgotten (Evernote is a great place to start). Because most popular recipes are born from available seasonal ingredients, there's a good chance you will find everything you need while shopping at the farmers market. If not, you might need to pick up the rest of your ingredients at a regular grocery store (this is not the end of the world).

10 Ways to Make Your Salad More Satisfying

I absolutely love salads, but if all you're eating is vegetables with a little bit of dressing, you won't get enough calories to keep you satisfied until your next meal. There are dozens of healthy additions you can use to make your salad more filling and delicious. Here are ten of my favorites.

1. Warm Ingredients

Grilled or sautéed onions, peppers, mushrooms, and meats wilt salad greens and make them slightly warm, adding depth and character to an otherwise boring salad.

2. Brown Rice

Adding a half cup of warm rice to a salad adds beautiful texture and flavor and keeps you full longer. Thawing one of your single-serving rice balls will add less than two minutes to your salad prep time.

3. Nuts

Walnuts, pistachios, and sliced almonds are my favorites, but feel free to try pecans, cashews, peanuts, pumpkin seeds, or anything else that sounds interesting.

4. Beans

Chickpeas, black beans, edamame, and other legumes are inexpensive and delicious ways to add some gravity to a salad.

5. Avocado

Half an avocado is sometimes exactly what a salad needs to take it to the next level.

6. Smoked Salmon

For a slightly more upscale salad experience, top your greens with a few slices of smoked salmon.

7. Quinoa

Mix in a small amount of quinoa as an accent or make it the base of a salad and then add cooked or raw vegetables and greens.

8. Grilled Meats

Your salad is a great place for summertime barbecue leftovers.

9. Egg

Boiled, fried, or poached, an egg is a wonderful way to make your salad more substantial.

10. Sardines

Canned fish is one of the easiest ways to get healthy protein and oils into your salad.

It is good to have a rough idea of when you are going to eat each of the meals you visualized. Some vegetables hold up better than others over the course of a week in the refrigerator, so you don't want to buy a boatload of squash blossoms if you aren't planning to use them in the next few days. Plan to eat the most delicate produce first, and save the hearty kale and broccoli for later in the week. Creative shopping without lists takes some practice, but you don't have to be a master chef or flavor expert to get it right. When cooking with delicious, seasonal ingredients, you can't go wrong with simplicity. Start with the basics and work your way up as you get more comfortable in the kitchen and at the market.

HOME COURT RECIPES

When learning to cook, focus on perfecting a few simple vegetable dishes and main courses that are simple and tasty. These will be your

Tips to Keep Produce Fresh

1. Shop regularly

It is probably self-evident, but it is still important to state that the freshest vegetables are the ones you bought today. They are even fresher if you get them at the farmers market (picked yesterday) rather than a grocery store that imports produce from around the world. In order to keep fresh vegetables and fruit in the house, shop for produce and groceries at least once a week.

2. Shop strategically

This is my true secret to keeping food fresh. Different foods have different shelf lives, and you can take advantage of this fact when planning your meals for the week. Always make sure you buy a few robust vegetables for your Thursday and Friday night dinners (or try to schedule your restaurant dates for later in the week).

Cruciferous vegetables (like broccoli, kale, collards, cabbage, chard, cauliflower, and brussels sprouts) and root veggies (including carrots, beets, parsnips, radishes, sunchokes, and potatoes) store the best and can last well over a week in the crisper (twist off the greens if they're still attached—most can be eaten, so feel free to save them and throw them in salads). Summer squash can last for many days in a dry plastic bag in the crisper, and winter squash can last weeks and sometimes months on a shelf. Eggplant has a shelf life similar to summer squash and can be stored in the same manner. Delicate vegetables like lettuce, spinach, and other spring greens are not as robust and should be eaten more quickly. Juicy fruits like berries, stone fruits, and even tomatoes are more time sensitive and should be incorporated into meals earlier in the week.

3. Cook intelligently

Having a rough idea of what meals you are going to make during the week can help you keep veggies fresh in several ways. In addition to planning your dishes around which vegetables last the longest, you can prepare large batches of food early in the week and then freeze or refrigerate the leftovers to eat later. Avoid overshopping by buying ingredients to use in multiple different dishes rather than buying extra items for vastly divergent menus. For example, rather than purchasing red peppers for a stir-fry and radishes for a salad, you can skip the radishes and add the extra pepper to your salad instead.

When buying herbs, I like to get one bunch of Italian parsley (it keeps a long time and is incredibly versatile) and only one bunch of a more delicate herb like thyme, dill, or cilantro. With this strategy you can explore recipes of different cuisines that utilize similar ingredients. For instance, if I have cilantro, I may make Mexican food one night and a Vietnamese dish another night. Both incorporate similar vegetables and herbs, but the flavor profiles of these cuisines are entirely different. This is where it comes in handy to have a well-stocked pantry—go beyond the basics and learn to work with ingredients like fish sauce, coconut milk, and anchovies. This is a great way to delve into a new cuisine and explore different flavors.

4. Store properly

Proper food storage can go a long way in keeping your produce as fresh as possible. Generally speaking, most vegetables maintain their crispness best in the aptly named refrigerator compartment, the crisper. Crispers have different humidity settings than the rest of the fridge and are optimized for vegetables. I find that leafy greens and herbs keep best in dry plastic bags or plastic storage containers. When you get home with a large bag of salad greens from the farmers market, rinse them clean and spin them in a salad spinner. Let them sit out for an hour or so to completely dry, and then put them in large plastic containers to store for the week. With this strategy the crisper is not necessary.

Most fruit I don't refrigerate to protect the taste, but berries are an exception. I have had fantastic luck storing berries in a jar or storage container with the lid closed tight. I always put my berries away immediately after getting them home, trying to handle them as little as possible to keep any mold or bacterial spores out. I try to roll the berries into their new container without actually touching them with my hands. I buy berries much more often now, since they don't go bad for me as quickly as they had in the past.

Finally, ripe fruits produce gases that cause neighboring fruits to ripen more quickly. If you have something that is perfectly ripe or over-ripe, you may want to keep it in the fridge away from the rest (unless of course you want the nearby fruit to ripen faster). Likewise, keeping fruits on the counter in paper bags will trap the gases and cause them to ripen more quickly if you want to speed up the process.

5. Don't give up

Sometimes despite your best efforts you end up with a wilted head of lettuce or a floppy bunch of basil. But if wilting is your only prob-lem and the plant looks otherwise edible (still green and free of mold), then all is not lost. The reason plants wilt is they lose water from their cells to the environment through osmosis. But the os-motic properties of leaves can be used to your advantage. You can revive wilted greens and even roots like carrots by submerging them in a bath of cold water for thirty to sixty minutes, which replenishes the water in the vegetables and allows them to regain their crisp-ness. It is astounding how much they will perk up.

Mold is another issue when storing fruits and vegetables, but you can sometimes salvage a batch of food if you catch it early and care-fully remove all traces of it to keep it from spreading to the rest of your produce (I recommend finding a new container for the uncontami-nated portion). Remember, mold is a living, growing thing that breeds more of itself. Keeping foods in sealed containers and touching them as little as possible with your hands can help control it.

default meals when you're feeling lazy and uninspired—your home court recipes. As your kitchen skills develop, you will surely explore recipes other than these, but having this base of easy, friendly recipes will make your transition to cooking at home much easier.

My lunchtime five-minute bean salad (Heirloom Bean Salad with Winter Vegetables, p. 221) is a perfect example of a home court recipe I turn to over and over again. I mix it up by switching out the seasonal

How to Make Cauliflower Taste as Good as French Fries

What's weird is that this is just roasted cauliflower; it couldn't sound any less glamorous. But for some reason roasting cauliflower completely transforms it from a vegetable people are pretty sure they don't like into something they just can't get enough of.

The coolest part of all is that anyone (like *any* anyone) can make this. I like to add curry powder to mine, but you can play around with whatever spices you like or just make it plain. (Pssst, try tossing in some fresh cilantro after it's done roasting.)

The trick is to use a very hot oven, around 500°. Covering the cauliflower for the first fifteen minutes steam-cooks it, while retaining the natural flavors and sugars. When you remove the foil the high heat browns and caramelizes the florets, giving the cauliflower a slightly crisp texture and complex flavor that is irresistible.

Cauliflower shrinks down substantially when cooked, and the biggest complaint I get from people about the recipe is that they wish they'd made more. It still freaks me out how good this is.

Roasted Curried Cauliflower
SERVES 2 TO 4

1 large cauliflower (or several small ones), about 2 pounds
Olive oil
Kosher or sea salt
Curry powder

Preheat the oven to 500°F (if you use a convection oven, 475°F may give you better results). Break the cauliflower head into medium-small florets and place them in a large bowl or baking pan. Be sure the pieces are as evenly sized as possible, or they will cook unevenly. The smaller you make the pieces, the quicker they will cook and the more caramelized they will become, which I consider a good thing.

Drizzle the cauliflower pieces generously with olive oil and season well with salt and curry powder. Distribute them evenly in a single layer on the bottom of a baking pan. If necessary, use a second baking pan to make sure the pieces aren't too crowded.

Cover the pans with foil and place into the oven. Roast, covered, for 10 to 15 minutes. The cauliflower should be slightly soft and start looking translucent. If it is not, replace the foil and roast another 5 minutes.

When the cauliflower has finished steaming, remove the foil and toss the florets with tongs. Continue to roast, stirring every 8 to 10 minutes until the tips of the cauliflower begin to brown and become crisp (don't be impatient; it's better if you wait until they're crispy), approximately 30 to 35 minutes.

herbs and vegetables, but the basic recipe is always the same. There are a few simple vegetable dishes I rely on frequently as well. My Roasted Curried Cauliflower is by far my most popular recipe, beloved by adults, children, and former cauliflower haters alike. The recipe is so simple even a newbie cook can get it right and convert an entire family into cauliflower lovers. You can rely on this recipe year-round whenever you're struggling to think of dinner ideas.

It's a good idea to have a small arsenal of green vegetables you can be confident about cooking up quickly and easily as well. Kale is one of my home court vegetables, and I typically make it by cooking it in olive oil on medium-high heat, with a little garlic and sea salt. If I have them around, I'll add some carrots, radishes, or nuts to make it a little more interesting, but it's tasty on its own. I prefer to use the red or purple kales, rather than the plain green curly kale. At certain times of year I use the darker Tuscan kale (dino kale or lacinato kale), which is easier to clean and chop.

Broccoli is another easy home court vegetable I turn to often. If possible I buy the smaller broccoli shoots rather than the large broccoli

Super Easy Kale with Pistachios

The key to making a plain green vegetable worthy of an entire meal is adding something with protein or fat (preferably both). Nuts work perfectly, as do any kind of beans or lentils. If you want to make your life even easier, look for kale with smaller, younger leaves so the stems are tender enough to cook and eat.

For me this meal is a perfect lunch. Alternately, you can serve it as a side dish for several people. If you would like a little more substance, serve it with lentils and brown rice or quinoa. I sometimes eat it with sardines, smoked mackerel, or trout on the side.

Sautéed Kale with Pistachios and Garlic
SERVES 1 TO 3

1 garlic clove
1 bunch kale (or chard)
¼ cup chopped pistachios (or other nut)
2 tablespoons extra-virgin olive oil
Sea salt to taste
½ cup cooked beans or lentils (optional)

Mince the garlic (letting your garlic sit 10 minutes after mincing increases its nutritional value). Rinse the greens and place them on a cutting board. It's okay if your greens are still wet; the water will help them steam. If you buy younger or smaller leaves, removing the stems isn't necessary. If the leaves have very thick stems, you may want to remove them by cutting them out or pinching the stem at the bottom and stripping off the leaves by running your hand along the spine.

Pile the leaves on top of each other all oriented in the same direction. Starting at the tip of the leaves, cut 1-inch strips until you have cut the entire bunch. If you are using Tuscan or red Russian kale, with thinner leaves, it will only need to be cut in this one direction. If your leaves are wide, cut them into 1- to 2-inch squares by making knife cuts in the opposite direction, parallel with the stem.

To a frying pan with tall sides and a lid, add the nuts and place it on medium heat. Lightly toast the nuts, stirring regularly with tongs. After 2 to 3 minutes, add the olive oil to the pan and allow it to heat up. Add the chopped greens to the pan, sprinkle generously with sea salt, and toss with tongs. Cover.

Stir the greens occasionally so they don't burn. Continue cooking the greens as they wilt and turn dark green. If they start to burn, lower the heat, add 1 to 2 tablespoons of water, and cover again to steam.

When the leaves are dark green and wilted, remove the lid and use tongs to toss, then clear a space in the center of the pan. Add the minced garlic in a single layer and cover with a small amount of additional olive oil. Allow the garlic to cook until it becomes fragrant, about 30 seconds, then mix it up with the kale and nuts. Add ½ cup of beans or lentils at this point, if desired.

Continue to cook greens uncovered for 1 or 2 more minutes. Taste-test a leaf and adjust salt to taste. Kale is done cooking when it is dark green and the stems are tender. Unlike spinach, it is very difficult to overcook kale, because it retains its crispness very well. Serve immediately.

crowns. I cut up all of it, leaves, stems, and all. Broccoli pairs beautifully with toasted cumin seeds and red chili flakes. Just toss in some garlic and a splash of rice vinegar at the end for a delicious side dish. Drizzle with some tahini to make it more filling.

Chard is another fantastic green that is available year-round. I cook it with sweet onions, pistachios, and mint leaves to brighten the flavor. It's also great with garlic. Chard has a natural salty taste, because it is so rich in potassium, so be careful not to oversalt it. It's also insanely good for you.

To change it up I also like to have a few red, orange, and yellow vegetables I cook regularly. I add sweet peppers and carrots to many dishes, but heartier vegetables like winter squash or sweet potatoes are great to have in your arsenal as well. I usually roast these because it concentrates the flavor and makes them taste amazing, but you could also pan-cook them in a bit of liquid and then blend them into a soup. Explore different vegetables and recipes until you find a few easy ones you like.

Similarly, it's nice to have a few easy fish, meat, or tofu/tempeh recipes you're comfortable making regularly. Roast chicken (Simple Roast Chicken, p. 105) is a fantastic meat to master, since leftovers can be used for days (another form of batch cooking) and the bones can be saved to use for chicken stock. In fact, any roast is fantastic for batch cooking, and a slow cooker is a great investment if you have a big family or enjoy having a lot of meat around to munch on. Salmon (wild Alaskan), shrimp, and halibut are all wonderful seafood options, and cooking them is incredibly simple. Just a few minutes in a pan on each side should do the trick. Adding a little salt, garlic, and lemon is an easy place to start, but play around with other flavors until you find some you enjoy.

DESSERT

Unless it's a special occasion, you probably shouldn't be eating dessert regularly at home, particularly if you're trying to lose weight. If you find yourself craving sweets at night, it's possible that your dinners are not satisfying enough. Try adding more starchy foods like beans, grains, or root vegetables to see if they decrease your cravings.

Fruit is an excellent option if you want a little something sweet and is often able to more than satisfy that nagging desire for sugar. I sometimes find that I'm more susceptible to sugar cravings if I've eaten something with a strong garlic or onion flavor. Fruit works wonderfully on these occasions, but often I just need to change the flavor in my mouth by brushing my teeth or having some mint tea. Herbal teas or

Better Than Butternut:
The Delectable Delicata Squash

Like most people, I hadn't heard of delicata squash before, but was a big fan of butternut. Butternut squash tastes rich and sweet and has a wonderful texture. It's also very filling and is a fantastic substitute for more starchy carbohydrates. But anyone who has tried to cook with butternut squash knows it isn't easy to work with. Butternut squash are huge, have a tough outer skin, and take longer than most vegetables to cook through. Lazy people don't cook butternut squash, and I came to accept the fact that I am one of those people.

Everything changed when I learned that not all winter squash require peeling. To me the difficult (and sometimes painful) peeling is the hardest part of cooking winter squash, so I was instantly intrigued about the possibility of alternatives. I was delighted to discover that the beautiful green Japanese "pumpkin" kabocha squash don't require peeling (woo-hoo!). I also discovered delicata.

Delicata are much smaller than most winter squash, making them substantially easier to get home from the market and more amenable to the needs of a small household. More important, delicata squash are a cinch to clean, cut, and cook, making them any winter squash lover's dream. Their flavor is even richer and their texture creamier than butternut.

I prefer to roast my delicata squash in a metal pan, allowing the outer edges to brown and caramelize. Although a Pyrex or ceramic pan will also work, I've found that I get better browning when I use a metal pan. Foil will give you a similar effect. The caramelization creates an almost sweet potato–like flavor. This is an all-time favorite winter home court recipe.

Roasted Delicata Squash
SERVES 2 TO 4 AS A SIDE DISH

2 to 4 delicata squash, depending on size (about 1½ pounds)
2 tablespoons olive oil
Salt to taste

Preheat the oven to 425°F. Clean the delicata squash by running them under warm water and scrubbing away dirt with a vegetable brush. If there are any hard spots on the squash, you can scrape them off with a butter knife.

With a sharp knife, cut the delicata in half lengthwise. This should be easy and not require any crazy hacking. With a spoon scoop out the seeds and discard (or save these and prepare them like pumpkin seeds if you wish).

Cut each delicata half into ½-inch segments, creating moon-shaped pieces that have slight bumps around the curve. Toss and coat the squash pieces in the olive oil, then arrange the pieces in a single layer in a metal baking pan. Too much oil can make the squash soggy. Salt gently. It's okay if the pieces are a little crowded, but try to maximize the surface area of the squash touching the pan. The browning only occurs where the squash and pan meet.

Place the pan in the oven and roast 10 minutes. Using a spatula (I use tongs for most veggies, but delicata squash are easily squished and hold up better if you don't pinch them), turn the squash in the pan so that the light sides are now touching the pan and the brown sides are facing upward.

Continue roasting, turning every 7 to 10 minutes until both sides of the squash pieces are golden brown and the texture is creamy to the teeth all the way through, about 25 to 30 minutes. Adjust salt. Serve as a side dish with the rest of your dinner.

tisanes are a delicious evening ritual that can sooth the nerves and tame cravings. Making these one of your home court habits might be your answer to ending those late-night splurges and saving your indulgences for when they're really worth it.

ELEVEN

THE OFFICE

Brown Bags and Bullies

"Stress is nothing more than a socially acceptable form of mental illness."
—RICHARD CARLSON, AUTHOR OF
DON'T SWEAT THE SMALL STUFF

"I have measured out my life with coffee spoons."
—T. S. ELIOT, *THE LOVE SONG OF J. ALFRED PRUFROCK*

"Time is an illusion. Lunchtime doubly so."
—DOUGLAS ADAMS, *THE HITCHHIKER'S GUIDE TO THE GALAXY*

For anyone with a day job, lunch at work is often the biggest challenge to eating healthier and losing weight. There is nary an office kitchen that isn't chock-full of junk food, from doughnuts and chips to sodas and Red Bull. Layer on hefty doses of stress and time pressure, and you have a recipe for a healthstyle disaster.

Even if you do manage to navigate the land mines of processed foods in the kitchen, limited facilities can mean there's no refrigerator or heating element, and what you bring from home is limited to what can be stored in your desk or shared space. Some office cultures create pressure to go out to restaurants, so bringing your own food can be seen as antisocial or, worse, a form of judgment on everyone else's eating habits. If your schedule is unpredictable, finding time to eat at all can be a challenge.

As hard as it is, finding a way to eat well at work is worth the effort. If you eat twenty-one meals during a typical week, almost a quarter of them will occur at the office. On the other hand, if you do manage to create a healthstyle that optimizes your workplace for health, it can put you well on your way to achieving your goals.

JUNK FOOD, JUNK FOOD EVERYWHERE

The number one complaint I hear from my readers is that their work environment is flooded with junk food. Organizations want to provide snacks for their employees, and by far the easiest and most affordable options are from big-ticket stores like Costco or Walmart, since they offer countless snack foods in bulk at rock-bottom prices. Health is rarely factored into the equation, and even if some healthy choices make it back to the office, they will likely to be accompanied by a lion's share of junk food to go around.

It's hard to blame anyone for this, since it is part of our culture. Most people grew up with and therefore like junk foods, so whoever makes these decisions at your company is surely just trying to make people happy by giving them what they want. Also, healthy foods tend to be more expensive and perishable, making them extremely inconvenient to stock unless a significant portion of employees will eat them (good luck with that). The end result is that almost everyone who works in an office is surrounded by free, convenient, and hyperpalatable food. For better or for worse, this aspect of your work environment is unlikely to change.

There are several things you can do to combat the allure of those sweet, sweet empty calories. The first step is changing the way you think about junk food. It may be free and convenient, but foodists recognize that processed foodlike substances aren't actually food, so on a typical weekday they should not be on the menu. Instead of telling yourself "I shouldn't" or "I can't" eat those generic boxed cookies, remind yourself, "As a foodist, I don't eat that way." In a series of studies published in the *Journal of Consumer Research,* scientist Vanessa Patrick and her team showed that saying "I don't" was almost three times more effective as saying "no" and eight times more effective than saying "I can't" in turning down food.[1] According to Patrick, "With 'I don't' you're choosing words that signal empowerment and determination rather than ones that signal deprivation," and that empowerment helps you make the right decision when faced with temptation.* Telling yourself that you don't drink calories, eat processed foods, or indulge in sweets at work is far more powerful than trying to convince yourself that you shouldn't. Patrick's team also showed that this strategy helps you make healthier decisions later on, empowering you to make better food choices even after you skirt the first temptation. In other words, how you think about unhealthy foods at work can boost your willpower at those times when you need it the most.

HEALTHY SNACKING 101

The next step in avoiding workplace junk food is having a healthy, reliable alternative ready to go. You can't expect a temporary bolstering of your willpower to last indefinitely, so having a snack food you can turn to when your stomach is trying to overpower your brain is absolutely necessary.

There's nothing wrong with snacking. Having a small bite to eat between meals is a great way to give your metabolism a little kick and keep you from becoming ravenously hungry later, which can lead to overeating. Snacking is also fun and can be a great way to socialize and

---

* By the way, this works for going to the gym as well. I, for one, don't skip workouts.

10 Reasons to Never Eat Free Food

Most people's eyes light up if free food is mentioned at work. But using the fact that something is "free" as an excuse to eat junk food is nothing to be proud of. We get excited by the concept of free food, because at first glance it seems like a good deal. But cheap, mass-produced food isn't worth much in health, taste, or even satisfaction. Thus one of the most important lessons I've learned in my twelve years of higher education is:

JUST BECAUSE IT'S FREE DOESN'T MEAN YOU HAVE TO EAT IT.

Occasionally someone will offer you high-quality food at no cost, but these opportunities are few and far between. More often you will find yourself wading through a sea of doughnuts, pizza, cookies, and other junk food. Your best bet is skipping the empty calories altogether when attending meetings, seminars, and other public events. Here's why.

1. It's cheap

You might think that free food is a bargain, but if you think about what you're really getting, it won't seem like such a good deal. Cheap food means low-quality, mass-produced calories made by industrial processes. That's the stuff we want to avoid.

2. It's flavorless

The right combinations of sugar, fat, and salt pretty easily deceive your brain, as these ingredients strongly activate your neural reward pathways. But if you try to focus on the true flavor of food and eat mindfully, you'll learn to taste the difference between real food and the flavorless industrial stuff.

3. It's bad for you

Processed foods are responsible for almost all "diseases of civilization," including heart disease, diabetes, and cancer. When you wolf down a few of those brownie bites at happy hour, you are directly contributing to your likelihood of developing these chronic diseases. Is that value?

4. You aren't saving money

You may tell yourself that this free meal will keep you from eating later, but there's a good chance you will eat again anyway. Processed foods do not satisfy you, but actually stimulate your appetite and strengthen future cravings. Also, if you factor in your future health-care costs, what you save by eating that $2 slice of free pizza starts to seem rather trivial.

5. You'll feel gross later

Junk food makes you feel bad, both physically and mentally. If someone offered you a free headache, would you take it?

6. It screws up your metabolism

Highly refined foods can induce insulin resistance over the next few hours, making both this and your next meal more fattening. If you make a habit of eating cheap abundant food, this condition can become chronic and develop into type 2 diabetes. What a bargain!

7. You'll gain weight

With insulin resistance comes weight gain, and with time you will gain more weight eating fewer calories. Unfortunately, people aren't often giving away free plus-size jeans.

8. You're eating empty calories

When you submit to eating cheap food, you are also choosing *not* to eat nutritious food. Choosing a diet rich in vitamins and other essential nutrients is necessary for reducing risk for sickness and disease, not to mention cravings. Foods typically offered as free don't even fulfill our most basic nutritional (or emotional) needs.

9. You don't need it

Chances are you get plenty of calories in your typical day. So why do you feel you need to eat junk food just because it is free?

10. It isn't worth it

The truth is free junk food isn't really free. Even if processed foods don't cost you money, they still cost you your health, happiness, and sense of well-being. As a foodist, you can do better.

connect with others. There is a difference, however, between snacking and compulsive, emotional, or hormonal eating. There is also a difference between snacking and bingeing.

No matter what your reason for snacking, the goal should always be satiation. If you are hungry, you want to eat enough to refocus your attention and avoid future overeating, and that's it. If you're snacking at a social event and aren't hungry, a few bites should be enough to get you chatting. If a midday hors d'oeuvre tastes amazing, a bite or two should satisfy your curiosity. If you're craving something, you want to stop the craving as quickly and effectively as possible.

Snacking should be a clearly defined occurrence, not something that drags out over the course of hours. It helps if your snacks come in fixed quantities to prevent mindless eating. When hunger is the issue, your goal should be to find snacks that are as healthy and satisfying as possible. Choose foods that are dense and digest slowly, so you feel as though you've eaten enough and aren't tempted to return for round two. Thinking about foods in terms of their macronutrients is rarely useful, but as a rule of thumb the most filling foods tend to have protein, fat, fiber, and water or some combination of these. Foods that have a lot of sugar or refined carbohydrates tend to do the opposite and encourage continual eating.

Cravings are a different beast and are the least awesome reason for snacking. They can be caused by nutrient deficiencies, hormone imbalances, or mental disquietude and can seem to come out of nowhere. Though giving into cravings sounds like a bad idea, attempting to ignore them can be distracting and often pointless.* So it is better to have a strategy for dealing with cravings rather than waste your time and energy putting off the inevitable. That said, cravings can often be alleviated without the specific food you think you want, so healthy options should always be your first resort. For instance, sugar cravings can often be eliminated with a piece of fruit, and a desire for calorie-dense, fatty foods can sometimes be quenched with a handful of trail mix. Even calorie-free beverages such as sparkling water and herbal tea can be effective.

---

* How long do you think you can ignore a food craving if the food you want is available? Yeah, I thought so.

Healthy Snack Ideas

Here are some snack ideas to get you started, but don't feel limited by this list. Start with foods you enjoy and work from there.

apples	charcuterie	boiled eggs
pears	sardines	sparkling water
melon	string cheese	tea
grapefruit	fancy cheese	tisane (herbal tea)
oranges	kale chips	
pistachios	carrots	dark chocolate
almonds	avocado	dried fruit
cashews	celery	mint tea
trail mix	bell pepper	juice spritzer
nut butter on fruit/veggie	zucchini	bean salad
smoked salmon	hummus	peanuts
jerky	edamame	yogurt
	lentils	

INSTAGRAM: A PARABLE

As much as we'd like them to, healthy snacks and lunches are un-likely to pack themselves. Enlightened organizations like Google take pride in supplying as many healthy treats as unhealthy ones for their employees, but the majority of us must fend for ourselves if we hope to stand a chance against the cookies and granola bars.* This poses a serious problem. When I polled my Twitter followers about the biggest challenges for eating healthy food at work, a popular tech writer replied with an answer that echoed what I heard from dozens of others: "All the reasons can be translated into this one sentence: 'I'm a lazy fuck.'" Planning ahead so that you have the resources to eat well on the job takes effort, and effort for distant goals like health and weight loss is more than a little hard to come by when work takes center stage.

To get a sense of what it takes to overcome these obstacles in a high-pressure office environment, I sat down with Instagram's founder, Kevin Systrom, and its first engineer, Shayne Sweeney. Instagram is a mobile application for taking and sharing photos that launched in October 2010. By December 2010, it already had one million registered users, and maintaining and scaling the app became the number one priority for the company's small team of five. "We never ate healthy at the release," recalled Systrom. "At least in the beginning, we'd be so into our work that crafting a salad out of arugula and radicchio just wasn't going to happen midday." Instead, they'd opt for the local food trucks or burritos near the office. Without their even realizing it, weight started to creep on:

"We were looking at old pictures from Instagram, and people were like, 'Oh my God, you look so young,' and I was like, 'What does that mean? Do I have gray hair? That was like six months ago,'" Systrom explained. "After that I kept telling myself, 'I've got to get healthy again,

---

* Don't kid yourself, granola bars are glorified candy.

I've got to get healthy again.' So I bought a scale one day and realized my weight was up to 235, and I had never been this heavy in my life. I used to be 210, and I was like, 'That's not okay.' But I knew I was not going to pull a sorority girl and just eat salad, because I love food. I can eat less, but I'm not going to stop eating food I like just to lose weight. That would make me unhappy."

For Sweeney the weight gain had an even deeper implication. "I had tipped the scale at 300 pounds five years ago, then lost 125 pounds. When I saw an interview I did a few months ago and I looked terrible, it was a big wake-up call. I knew I could get to a point where I was incredibly unhealthy, so I had this motivation. I thought back and tried to remember what I was doing when I lost weight before. Exercise was the first thing we talked about, so Kevin and I went back to running," recalled Sweeney. The two started waking up a half hour earlier each morning and running on the treadmill at the gym. "It was hard for the first three weeks, but then it got really addictive," said Systrom. "We'd compare how many calories we burned at the end of it, and I realized you could actually map how much you exercise to how many calories you burn."

Healthy eating came as a direct result of this observation. "What's interesting is we started with exercise, but we were seeing results by understanding that you spend this amount of time and you burn this many calories, so we would make a conscious effort to eat healthier," Sweeney recounted. "We didn't go into it with the mindset of dieting." Systrom agreed. "Now I get angry when I see someone eating greasy potato chips, because I know that is a forty-minute run, and a forty-minute run is hard. So eating healthy was a consequence of starting to exercise."

Once healthy eating became a priority, convenience and foresight became the name of the game. Systrom found that stocking yogurt in the office fridge and picking up soups and precut carrot sticks from Whole Foods was the secret to staying on track. "The key for me was finding tricks so you're not starving, but also so you enjoy eating healthy. I love Greek yogurt, because it fills me up, and the stuff is so good!" he explained excitedly. "I just had stuff around so that when I was hungry and angsty for food, I knew where to go, instead of going to the cupboard and getting chips."

Sweeney's strategy included opting for the vegetarian lunch from the Instagram caterer. "During the week, I only eat vegetarian. It isn't because I have anything against meat. It just seems like the vegetarian option on everything that comes in is more healthy," he told me.

Systrom doesn't take it this far, but makes a point to load up on veggies and eat them first before allowing himself a smaller, more indulgent treat that he really enjoys. Both agree that it comes down to value. "To me, lunch at work is nothing special," said Sweeney. "To go waste a ton of calories and go get a crappy burrito from around the corner makes no sense. I'd rather spend my weekends or one night a week going to a great restaurant where there's great food."

Systrom and Sweeney began changing their healthstyle in May 2012, shortly after Facebook announced its plans to acquire Instagram for $1 billion. Before this time they didn't worry much about what they ate, particularly Systrom, who considers restrictive dieting to be far too difficult in a startup environment. "It's so painful. You get to work and you can't think. The way we eat now is way more fulfilling," he said. Sweeney would occasionally try a restrictive diet, but these temporary diversions never made much of a difference. "I once did this juice thing where I didn't eat at all for a week. It was terrible," he shared with a tinge of regret. But things are different now. "I don't feel cheated at lunch. I find things that I like, and I realized, 'Wow, I actually like vegetarian options.' And I don't feel guilty on the weekends when I go have a great dinner."

Finding time to exercise turned out to be easier than they expected. They realized that they had to work out in the mornings, since their availability in the evenings was inconsistent. So in the beginning they forced themselves to get up earlier and hit the gym. "The truth is you have to give up something. I give up sleep and a little bit of morning work time, and I'm okay with that," Systrom said. But he went on to explain that what they lose in time, they gain in efficiency, since their morning workouts make them more alert. "I get in about thirty minutes later, but I'm so much more productive and can stay later," said Systrom. The only time their productivity took a hit was in the early weeks when they weren't yet adapted to the morning workouts. According to Systrom, "It wasn't that easy the first three weeks, but I made a deal with myself that if it still sucked after four weeks, I would stop. But it didn't. It was great." Despite getting to work a half hour later and losing out on a little sleep that the lazier versions of themselves would relish, their new habits help rather than hinder their work. "We're actually much more productive in the mornings now," Sweeney agreed. "Having the structure was actually better all around."

Systrom believes that his newfound confidence in how he looks and feels also plays a big role in his increased productivity. "I feel way more energetic, but I think that's because I'm more confident. I've lost twenty-five pounds now,* and people say 'Wow, you look good!'" He paused briefly as he glanced down at himself, then over to Sweeney. "We can tuck our shirts in finally. Seriously, I can fit into a large now and not the bulky extra large, and that felt really good. And because of that I think I'm more energetic at work."

In the beginning, before they started seeing results and when waking up earlier was still really hard, there were two things that kept them motivated. "The only reason I was doing it was because we were doing it together. We stopped going to the gym together after a month, but it was necessary in the beginning," Systrom explained. "I don't think anyone should have to do it alone. It's just really hard." As mentioned in chapter 8, finding the motivation to exercise consistently should be your top priority when starting a new workout regimen. Once you

---

* It had been three months at the time of this interview.

reach a certain level of fitness, exercise becomes its own reward, but before that workouts can be painful and you need to find a way to push through those first few weeks. "If you find a buddy, you keep each other motivated," continued Systrom. "Social accountability actually matters, and for us it just meant showing up."

The second big motivator for Systrom and Sweeney was having a way to quantify and share their progress with friends. "Nike+ was awesome for us, because you see how many calories you burn and how long you go. It's infectious too. My girlfriend started running every day," said Systrom. Modern electronic activity trackers allow you to both follow your progress and share that information with friends, even if you don't work out with them directly. Being able to see your friends' activity becomes a form of inspiration and motivation. "It's not a competition in an aggressive sense," Sweeney explained. "You get addicted to it, and it becomes fun. We continue to encourage each other."

Systrom believes these subtle psychological motivators are what enabled him and Sweeney to overcome the barriers that make healthy living so difficult in an office environment. "You can't trust yourself in difficult situations. You have to set yourself up for success," he says. "Changing small, contextual things in your life completely changes the game." Tiny actions have the power to change whether you view a task as doable or difficult, and harnessing this power to help you build healthy habits is the key to achieving results. These actions can be as simple as bringing in yogurt and soup for lunch, sharing with your friends on Nike+, or packing your gym bag before going to bed. "I knew that if I didn't pack my gym bag with the clothes I was going to wear the next day, I wouldn't make it to the gym. I also needed to lay out my workout clothes. I'd wake up in the morning and just make myself a deal: 'Listen Kevin, all you need to do is put on those clothes and you'll wake up on the drive to work and you'll be fine.' Everything is set up for me. But if it's too much work to get up in the morning, you won't do it," he reflected. "There have been times when I have literally considered sleeping in my running clothes, so all I'd have to do is get up and put on my shoes."

The same is true of food. "Preparation is so key. It's all about doing things before you get hungry, because once I get hungry I make irrational decisions," Systrom continued. "You don't want to be thinking when you're panicking, and hunger is a form of panic." Habit usually compels people to choose the most convenient foods when they suddenly find themselves hungry, which is almost never the healthiest or tastiest option. Having an easy, tasty, and healthy alternative is the secret to overriding this impulse. "You need to train yourself to have certain reactions in specific situations. When you get hungry just do this, this, and this, and if you just follow those, it all gets better really quickly. But if you panic, you just go get a burrito. Game-time decisions are never good."

At Instagram, Systrom and Sweeney developed a set of rewarding healthstyle habits that led to rapid and relatively painless results. For most people, the biggest fear in integrating healthy habits into their work life is that it will take up too much time and energy and that their productivity will go down as a result. The team at Instagram proves that this does not have to be the case and that the benefits of upgrading your healthstyle more than justify the initial investment. Moreover, if your job is the main focus of your attention and you're spending more than forty hours per week in a work environment, your results may be even more profound than those for someone who spends less time at the office, since a larger proportion of your weekly habits will be promoting good health. "The best thing about this was seeing results—seeing weight go down was awesome, and that's what kept me going," said Systrom. Working long hours takes enough of a toll on your quality of life; it shouldn't negatively impact your physical well-being as well. You owe it to yourself to stop finding excuses and start finding ways to integrate healthy living into your work life.

THE BUDDY SYSTEM

An essential component of Systrom and Sweeney's success came from their simple decision to start on their journey together. Since the hardest part of upgrading your healthstyle is the first few weeks when your new habits are not yet formed, having a partner who keeps you motivated and accountable can be the difference between success and failure. In an office environment, however, having a buddy for support can have a profound social impact as well.

I've had many people complain to me that one of the most difficult aspects of changing their habits at work is the social pressure put on them by their coworkers who don't value health. Healthy eaters are often subject to ridicule and pressured to abandon healthy habits in favor of less healthy ones. In these situations, having a friend who is making healthy changes with you is particularly valuable. Social dynamics completely change when you're doing something as a group instead of on your own. Instead of being an outlier, you are a team member and your actions are viewed as different instead of just weird. Even if some of your coworkers continue to mock your choices, at least you have the support of someone else to stick to your guns and do what you know is best.

In talking to Systrom and Sweeney I was taken aback by the lack of blowback they experienced from colleagues. "It has actually been pretty neat. It started with just the two of us doing the vegetarian option and eating healthier, and now the vegetarian option counts for over a third of our office's lunch order, because people want to eat a little healthier," said Sweeney.

A few people in the office joined their gym as well. "It's infectious, and people around you start to notice. People catch on. Everybody wants to be healthy and look good, feel good," he continued. Whether their coworkers would have been so enthusiastic if only one of them had started making changes is less clear. "I think everyone wants to eat healthy, but when they see other people doing it, it seems kind of cool. Like a trend," Systrom explained. Having more than one person involved makes creating healthy habits a cultural shift rather than a lone mission.

SALAD CLUB

When you recruit colleagues to join in your foodist adventure, a world of possibilities opens up. E. Foley, copywriter and creator of the geek-centric dating site GeeksDreamGirl.com, developed a potluck-style salad bar at her office that she calls Salad Club.

The first rule of Salad Club is to recruit as many members as possible. Foley was able to wrangle eight of her coworkers into participating. She created a shared spreadsheet on Google Docs and has members commit to bringing one or two salad ingredients for the week. On Monday, everyone brings in their goods and puts them in the office fridge. Then every day at lunch members can dig into the ingredients and create the salad of their choice.

A Salad Club has tremendous benefits. One of the best is that eating a healthy lunch requires almost no effort or planning. You just need to go get the ingredients you are bringing and remember to take them with you on Monday. Lunch for the rest of the week is then taken care of. Another benefit is that you can try new vegetables and ingredients without committing yourself to an entire week's worth of something you may not like. Similarly, bringing in a few of your own items ensures that there will be at least something there you enjoy.

Also, if you have enough people participating, Salad Club makes it possible to eat something different every day. It will always involve healthy food, but you can mix and match flavors, so you never need to eat the same thing twice. Finally, Salad Club creates a social lunch experience that is far more cost-effective than spending several days a week going out with the crew. Foley explained that with Salad Club she spends less on food for the week than she typically spends on a single lunch when she goes out to a restaurant with coworkers.

Salad Club is an excellent example of using the buddy system to overcome typical office obstacles to healthy eating. It makes healthy choices convenient, fun, delicious, and affordable. And if renaming your lunch hour Salad Club gives you extra inspiration by reminding you of a shirtless Brad Pitt with rippling abs, so much the better.* The only other thing you need to remember is that if this is your first time at Salad Club, you have to eat.

PLANES, TRAINS, AND CONFERENCES

Keeping work hours healthy can be especially difficult if traveling is a big part of your job. The quality of food at most airports rivals even the grossest of elementary-school cafeterias,† and things rarely improve once you nestle into your business-class window seat. It's not just the unhealthiness of airport and airplane food that's upsetting. Adding insult to injury, the food is disgusting. As Tim Ferriss, author of *The 4-Hour Chef*,[2] once eloquently tweeted, "Each time I eat airport food, a small part of my soul dies." Airport and airplane food is neither healthy nor delicious, which means none of those empty calories are worthy of a foodist's indulgence.†† Finding alternatives requires a little planning and foresight, but the effort is more than worth it.

Step one in avoiding airport food is not being hungry when you get to the airport. This may sound obvious, but in my experience few people bother to plan for a proper meal while preparing for travel, and this is a fatal mistake. Making sure you eat something substantial be-

---

*No, this is not sexist. Both men and women alike have reason to be impressed with those serratus muscles.

† There are certainly some exceptions; the Virgin America Terminal 2 at SFO is amazing.

†† Never forget that everything unhealthy *is* an indulgence, whether you like it or not.

fore waiting in the security line can get you through a flight of up to six hours with little more than a snack. In contrast, skipping the meal virtually dooms you to at least one subpar dining experience for any flight over three hours.

What you eat before you fly doesn't have to be time-consuming or complicated, but it does have to be filling. If all you can find the time for is some quick scrambled eggs or a cup of yogurt with muesli, that's still light-years better than a two-day-old salad or plastic-wrapped sandwich you'll likely find at the airport. If you have time for an even more substantial meal, that's fantastic. But five minutes is really all it takes to get you through your flight with minimal suffering.

The next step in avoiding airplane food is bringing adequate meals and snacks. I rely heavily on nuts and trail mix for both short and long flights. They're compact, nonperishable, relatively healthy, and pleasantly filling in a pinch. If you bring your own, you will have your favorites, but if you forget them, it is possible to find packs of almonds, cashews, or peanuts in the airport. Other useful, portable snacks include hard fruits like apples or oranges (though be careful if you're flying across borders), jerky, string cheese, boiled eggs, and nori (crispy seaweed).

When traveling on longer flights I often bring entire meals to get me through without relying on the airline food service. Grain salads are particularly amenable to transport, since they are just as tasty at room temperature as they are fresh out of the fridge. They can be eaten on their own or used as a supplement to the better items the airline provides. Rather than preparing and packing a special meal on the day of your flight, you might want to make a large batch of farro or quinoa salad for lunch or dinner the day before the trip and then pack up the leftovers in a disposable container. When it's time to go to the airport, you can just grab it on your way out the door and eat it at your convenience.

Unfortunately, sometimes eating in an airport or on a plane is in-evitable. Maybe your flight is delayed, maybe your flight is super long, maybe you packed your food but ran out the door without it. It happens.

Flight-Friendly Food

Mexican-Style Quinoa Salad

SERVES 2 TO 3

1 cup dry quinoa
½ cup chopped red pepper
1 green onion or shallot, chopped
½ cup grape tomatoes, halved
1 clove garlic, minced
½ cup chopped cilantro
2 tablespoons olive oil
Half bag of arugula or baby spinach
Salt and cayenne pepper
1 lime
Tapatio or favorite Mexican hot sauce

Rinse and cook the quinoa in excess water until tender, 10 to 15 minutes. While the quinoa is cooking, cut up the pepper, onion, and tomatoes, mince the garlic, and chop up the cilantro, stems and all. If you are using a green onion, save some for garnish.

When the quinoa is finished cooking, drain and set it aside. Heat a frying pan on medium-high heat and add the olive oil. Add the onions and red peppers and cook until caramelized, about 10 minutes. Add the garlic and cook until fragrant, about 30 seconds. Turn off the heat and add the quinoa, stirring to mix. Fold in the arugula or spinach and season with salt and cayenne pepper to taste.

Transfer the quinoa mixture to a large serving bowl and add the tomatoes and cilantro. Squeeze in the juice of half a lime, add a few dashes of Tapatio or other hot sauce to taste, and stir. Adjust salt and spices. Garnish with green onion slices, extra cilantro leaves, and a wedge of lime. Store leftovers in disposable containers in the fridge.

Eating in an airport every once in a while won't kill you, and there are a few tricks you can use to minimize the damage. Your number one goal should be to find simple food. I've mentioned nuts, but I also sometimes look for boiled eggs, vegetable and fruit salads, and other foods in which I can identify all the ingredients by eye. Mexican food is often a good choice, since you can typically find beans, rice, salsa, and simple grilled vegetables and meats. I love a good pizza, but would never eat it at an airport, since it's probably filled with industrial dough conditioners and overly processed mystery cheese and meat.

On the plane I sometimes opt for the vegetarian, gluten-free, or diabetic meals. This will typically result in more vegetables, less industrial meat, and fewer flour-based foods. I often do this at conferences as well when I know the food won't taste very good and I want it to be as healthy as possible. Be careful, though, if you do plan to go with the vegetarian option; you may want to double-check with the organization (or flight attendant) beforehand to see that you aren't trading down for pasta, which won't score you any points in the health game.

FAST FOODIST

The other big issue when traveling for work is the lack of a kitchen. At home, a small amount of planning on weekends can easily set you up for healthy snacks and meals the rest of the week. But on the road, healthy eating is a bit more challenging.

When staying in a hotel for work in another city, the first thing I look for is a Whole Foods or other health-food store that is likely to have a decent selection of healthy snacks.* If they have a deli or prepared-food section, this is my first choice for quick, healthy meals, a foodist version of fast food. Alternately, organic cafés or specialty

---

* Protip: I do this when visiting family too.

vegetarian or vegan restaurants are usually a reliable source for real, unprocessed foods. Plugging terms like "organic," "natural foods," "whole foods," "vegetarian," and "vegan" into Google maps can open a world of possibilities. Although I don't think eating vegetarian or even organic is necessary to be healthy, these terms filter out a lot of the industrial stuff we're looking to avoid and are a useful hack for finding healthy food in an unfamiliar city.

In general, if you spend a lot of time on the road for work, you need to become an expert in finding stores and restaurants that specialize in whole, unprocessed foods. You must also master the art of navigating restaurant menus and portions, which we cover in chapter 12. Finally, don't be too hard on yourself. You should certainly do your best to eat healthy whenever possible, but occasionally it won't work out and you'll be stuck eating something you would have rather avoided. So long as this doesn't become a habit, it's not the end of the world.

TWELVE

RESTAURANTS

The Good, the Bad, and the Ugly

"One of the very nicest things about life is the way we must regularly stop
whatever it is we are doing and devote our attention to eating."
—LUCIANO PAVAROTTI

"In life, as in restaurants, we swallow a lot of indigestible stuff
just because it comes with the dinner."
—MIGNON MCLAUGHLIN, *THE NEUROTIC'S NOTEBOOK*, 1960

Eating in restaurants means different things to different people. For
some it's a rare opportunity to go out and celebrate life's great mile-
stones. For others it's a way of life. I pity the fool who puts health over
pleasure every time he or she enters a restaurant. Great food is like great
art, and the experience is often worth looking past carbs and calories
for the sake of living life. Foodists have already budgeted for the occasional guilt-free splurge anyway.

If you eat out often, however, too many dips into the bread basket will
quickly size you out of your favorite jeans. Knowing when to say when
at restaurants is one of the most difficult healthstyle skills to develop, but
if restaurants are more than a casual hobby for you, then it is essential.

Tackling restaurants like a foodist requires an intimate understanding of your own healthstyle and values. We already know we can't rely on willpower to force ourselves into smart decisions, so it helps to have a strategy that accounts for all the factors that are important to our health and happiness. That way, when we're faced with the choice, we already have a plan of action.

THE DINER'S DILEMMA

Some problems with restaurants are universal. Even when the ingredients are listed on the menu, you are rarely warned about all the butter, cream, oils, bread crumbs, sugar, and other hidden ingredients that make food yummy and decadent. Not that you need to actively avoid these ingredients if you like them, but it is important to remember that they are very rich and add a huge number of calories to a meal that might otherwise sound light and healthy. Predicting what exactly will arrive after you place your order is difficult, and once it's in front of you resisting temptation is even harder. Thus one of the most important strategies for avoiding overeating in restaurants is focusing on the things you can control, such as eating slowly and mindfully.

Rare is the eating establishment that doesn't serve portions fit for a king. Most of us could stop at 75 percent of what we're served and still consume far more than we need to be satisfied. Since we're so bad at judging large portion sizes, few of us even realize how much restaurants cause us to overeat. There are a few ways to handle this issue. One solution is to simply stop eating, though this may be easier said than done. As one of my very slender friends explained to me, "People just need to get over the guilt of leaving food on their plate when they're no longer hungry."

We are naturally wired to finish our plates, no matter how big. When I was growing up, my mom always told me that I needed to eat everything I was served, because children in other countries were starving. Of course, she never bothered to explain why our family's gluttony made everything okay in the rest of the world. Nothing good happens from you stuffing yourself, and if it really bothers you, go ahead and mail your leftovers to the other side of the planet. Better yet, take what you don't eat in a doggy bag and make another meal of it or offer it to a hungry person on the street. The key point to understand is that, since restaurant portions are absurdly large, you need to train yourself to stop eating when full or close to full.

Once you've convinced yourself you don't need to clean your plate, the challenge becomes stopping yourself before all the food is gone, because, let's face it, tasty food is tasty. There are a few effective strategies that can help. First, research has repeatedly shown that people get more pleasure from the first bite of food than any other. With this in mind, start your meal by eating the best things on your plate rather than saving them for last. That way when you start to feel full, it is much easier to set your fork aside, since you know you've already had the most delicious bite. Another way to avoid the oversize-portion trap is to get in the habit of sharing plates. It feels unnatural at first, but once you try it, you'll see that you can share most dishes with a dining partner and still get plenty of food; this holds for men as well as women. If you really want your own entree, chances are you don't need anything else on the menu, such as an appetizer or dessert.

At restaurants, the only thing worse than jumbo portions is the bread basket. Premeal bread is the worst. Not only does it contain some of the most useless calories in the human diet; it tortures and taunts you while you're waiting for the food you've already decided is worth your time and calories. More often than not, I choose to skip it altogether. If you can't handle the basket sitting on the table, explain to the server that you don't need any bread. If you're trapped because everyone else at the table is on a dinner-roll feeding frenzy, distract yourself by ordering a good drink and striking up conversation. As I explained in chapter 2, the bread basket is one of the few places I still need to exercise willpower in my healthstyle, but I never regret it when I do.

That restaurants frequently course meals is another reason they encourage overeating. When plates and plates of amazing looking and smelling foods are placed in front of you, who wouldn't want to try everything? Variety may be the spice of life, but it's also a great way to eat more than you should. Avoid this by ordering less. Ask your server how many plates are appropriate for your party, and assume that's at least 20 percent more than you need (i.e., drop a small plate). It's easier to have restraint briefly and order less than to rely on willpower to restrain yourself when all that food shows up on your table. You can always order more if you find it isn't enough, but this will rarely be the case.

Alcohol is another reason it's tough to have restraint at dinner. Even as devout foodists brimming with willpower, we need to exercise restraint at most restaurants worth eating at, given how much extra food we are confronted with. The problem is that the source of willpower is the frontal lobes of our brains, and alcohol is notorious for shutting these down. Another issue is the significant amount of extra sugar and calories in the drinks themselves. Although a glass of wine or spirits won't do much damage, a margarita or other sweet cocktail contains hundreds of calories, mostly sugar. Just think of it as dessert in a glass. As obvious as it sounds, drinking less can really help.

A good friend in the restaurant business recently introduced me to the "half cocktail," which is basically half the size (and sugar/alcohol content) of a regular cocktail. The half cocktail is brilliant, because you get the pleasure of trying some wonderful drinks, but the damage done by the calories and booze is a fraction of what it could be. This might not be an official option at the bar, but it is certainly a possibility at home or if you're out with a close friend with the same taste in drinks.

If drinking less is really hard for you, try ordering drinks with less alcohol and sugar. European wines, for example, tend to have less alcohol than big California wines. Similarly, white wines contain less alcohol than red wines. On the flip side, Belgian beers can have nearly as much alcohol as a bottle of wine, so lighter domestic beers are often

8 Tips for Drinking Less Without Your Friends Knowing

I have nothing against people who like to party. Partying is really fun, and a lot of the time I'm right there leading the crusade. But we all know those people who *really* like to drink, and like to do it often. Not only do these people take their own drinking a little too far; they're experts at pressuring others to keep up with them drink for drink. And they'll use mockery, guilt, generosity, logic, peer pressure, and dozens of other tactics to get everyone around them to keep the party going. These friends are fun to have, until they aren't. As fun as it is to party, sometimes you want to go out and have a good time without regretting it the next day. Rejecting drinks can be even more awkward if alcohol is a big part of your offsite work culture, where turning down a glass makes you look antisocial or not a team player. It is nice to have a way to hit it a little less hard, preferably without drawing attention to your secret plan. Feel free to mix and match these tricks, as different situations call for different lines of defense.

1. Alternate with water

Alternating with water is a tried-and-true way to both cut back on alcohol and stay hydrated, thereby preventing a hangover. Every drink or two, go to the bar and ask for some water. You don't need to make excuses for this: you're thirsty and will get another drink in a second. Just be sure to finish the water and feel free to take your time.

2. Drink clear liquids

Clear liquids like gin and vodka look like ice that has melted. So if you don't want to finish every drink that comes your way, you can always leave a little in your old glass, and no one will notice you aren't tossing back as much as everyone else is.

3. Order drinks that look like alcohol (but aren't)

Another advantage of clear liquids. Vodka soda with lime is my favorite go-to drink on late nights, and it's awesome for several reasons.

Besides being easily palatable and sugar free, it gives you the option of leaving out the vodka altogether. Just order a club soda with lime and ask the bartender to make it look like a cocktail—they are usually more than happy to comply.

4. Be forgetful

You don't have to be limited to clear liquids to abandon the occasional half-full glass. Leave your drink on the bar, in the bathroom, on a random table, or anywhere it won't attract attention. That way when someone hands you another, you're ready.

5. Drink light beer

If you're a beer drinker and all this talk of clear liquid is making you squirm, never fear. There is a huge difference in the alcohol content of beers, with light beers coming in around 4 percent alcohol and some fancy Belgians topping out at over 10 percent. You do the math.

If you know you'll have to get through more than you've bargaining for, opt for lighter beers. If you're like me and think some domestic light beer tastes like donkey pee, go with a Mexican beer like Corona and add a lime. I can drink those all night and barely get a buzz going—and I'm little.

6. Master the shot spit

Drinking nights often don't turn crazy until someone starts ordering shots, and then it's all over. Bartenders have this problem too, since drunk people often think they've found a new best friend and gratefully buy their server shots throughout the night. To avoid getting hammered on the job, bartenders keep a half-empty pint of beer nearby and pretend to use it as a chaser when in reality they are spitting the shots back into it.

If you know your friends are likely to "surprise" everyone with shots, be sure to have a nearby water glass or pint that you're nursing. Use the old bartenders' trick, and no one will suspect. I know it's gross, but it works. Just remember to not actually drink the beer later.

7. Show up late

Sometimes special occasions are specifically set aside for excessive drinking. If you need to make an appearance, but would rather not sacrifice your liver, show up forty-five minutes to an hour late. Everyone else will already be one drink ahead of you.

8. Order half shots

If you're in charge of ordering your own drinks and vodka soda isn't your thing, ask for your regular cocktail, but request a half shot instead of a normal one. You'll still get the fun of drinking, but each drink will contribute less to tomorrow's headache.

a better choice. If wine and beer aren't your thing, there are plenty of amazing cocktails that don't require added sugar. Talk to your bartender to find the best options for you. Another great strategy is alternating between alcoholic drinks and water. This will both prolong your evening stamina and temper tomorrow's head pain. Choose your drinks wisely to find that perfect balance of fun and foresight.

Finally, dessert is far more likely than not to be offered if you're eating at a restaurant. It's your call if the restaurant is good enough or the occasion is special enough to justify the order. Sometimes it will certainly be worth it. Remember, though, that to dessert or not to dessert is not the only question. Even on special occasions you shouldn't pretend that ten bites is the same as four. Desserts typically run 25 to 75 calories *per bite,* and extras really do matter. If you don't need to finish it, you probably shouldn't. Sharing makes this much easier.

YOUR CALL

You can solve a lot of the difficulties of restaurants if you have a say in choosing the spot. Whenever possible, volunteer to do the planning, so you have better options. We're in the midst of a food revolution, and it's getting easier to find places that focus on real, local, and seasonal ingredients. These should be your top choices if they're in your budget. Because high-quality food is typically more expensive than mediocre industrial food, expect these restaurants to be a little pricier than a standard chain restaurant. They aren't all prohibitively expensive though, and if you look hard enough, you can often find some real gems.

There are a few ways to identify foodist-friendly restaurants. The most obvious is their emphasis on ingredients. People who make the effort to source excellent food are never shy about the extra work they've put in. A restaurant's philosophy will often be featured prominently on its website or menu. If the ingredients for a dish also mention the farm from which the ingredients were sourced, this is an excellent sign. Similarly, great ingredients tend to be seasonal, and restaurants that focus on local, seasonal products frequently change their menu to reflect this. People who take pride in their work create better products than people just looking to turn a profit. These are the places you want to eat at when given the choice.

LA VIDA LOCAL

City life brings lots of options, but most of us gravitate to a few favorite spots for the sake of convenience and familiarity. Sometimes nothing is better than sinking into a booth at your favorite local haunt and ordering the dish you're convinced is the best of its kind in the city. I love the burger at my secret neighborhood spot more than most other foods on earth, but if I ordered it every time I visited, it wouldn't be pretty. At the places you eat at often, it's just as important to find something healthy you enjoy on the menu as it is to find that decadent indulgence that makes you melt, because you can't splurge every time without consequences. On the other hand, if you eat mostly at home and only go there every now and again, you can eat whatever you want. You need to figure out for yourself what your healthstyle budget can absorb. I indulge my burger habit once every month or so, and it is glorious. Thankfully, the healthy dishes on the menu are just as amazing.

Healthier choices are not always easy to find at restaurants. At places I eat at often, I'm not shy about making special requests and substitutions. This sometimes means ordering salads without croutons, leaving the rice out of my burrito, or asking for vegetables instead of potatoes. They don't all work at every spot, and I don't make the change if I feel it will severely and negatively impact my enjoyment of the dish. But if I'm just as happy with oil and vinegar on my salad as I am with the honey-glazed syrup that is normally used, then I don't hesitate to ask for it. At the very least I try to make sure there is something green on my plate every time I eat. Adding colorful vegetables brightens any meal, and people often look at my plate with envy when we've ordered the same thing, but mine shows up with a vibrant salad instead of a pile of soggy fries.

Remember too that choosing salad doesn't always mean you have to skip the fries completely. When I eat with friends, there is almost always someone else who would prefer to eat healthier, but would also love to try a few fries. See if anyone wants to go splitsies with you on the dishes (e.g., I'll get the lasagna and you get the spinach salad), or go in on an extra order of fries "for the table." That way you get to try them, but don't eat the entire basket, and you still get your share of greens. Everyone's a winner.

Keep a mental (or physical, if you're still journaling) record of how often you splurge and how it affects you. I find that one or two delicious-but-coulda-been-healthier meals can fit into my weekly healthstyle budget fairly easily, but many more than that can make my pants start to feel tighter. When you count your indulgences, it forces you to question whether you're making the right decision in the moment and to ask yourself if this particular meal is worth sacrificing for a better option later in the week. This mindfulness alone is often powerful enough to keep you on the right track.

10 Simple Substitutions for Making Restaurant Foods Healthier

When nothing on the menu perfectly fits my preferences, I don't hesitate to swap out whatever I don't want for something better. Whether it's to avoid processed foods or simply add vibrance and color to your plate, here are ten simple swaps to make the most of your restaurant meals.

1. Mixed greens instead of iceberg or romaine lettuce

I enjoy Cobb salads, but for some reason they're usually made using old iceberg lettuce. Most places these days carry mixed greens or spinach as well and are usually happy to make the switch.

2. Fruit instead of toast

I'm not sure why breakfast spots think you need two giant pieces of toast on top of your potatoes, eggs, and pancakes, but if you don't want toast, they'll often offer you fruit instead. This is one of the best upgrades you can get away with.

3. Salad instead of potatoes

Speaking of potatoes, although they are real food and have their place in a healthy diet, they're so often fried in rancid industrial oils that it's best to skip them. Swapping them out for salad or cooked greens is rarely a problem.

4. Avocado instead of mayo

Real mayonnaise, the kind made from egg yolks and olive oil, is perfectly healthy (and delicious). Unfortunately, that isn't what most places are putting on your sandwich. Instead, commercial mayos are typically made with soybean or canola oil (i.e., overprocessed industrial oil). It may cost a little extra, but avocado is a fantastic alternative to gooey up your lunch.

5. Cheese plate instead of dessert

One of the things I love about France is that it's perfectly acceptable to have cheese after dinner instead of sugar. If everyone is ordering crème brûlée and you don't want to be a party pooper, get the cheese plate instead. Good cheese is healthy.

6. Brown rice instead of white

I don't mind white rice in small quantities, but if I'm stuck eating somewhere where I know the food isn't very healthy, I'll swap out my white rice for brown (and order as many vegetables as possible) if the option is available.

7. Wine instead of cocktails

Dinner often starts with a drink selection. Although wine certainly has calories, cocktails usually have hundreds more thanks to the liqueurs and syrups typically used. Mixed drinks have their place, but if you'll also be eating an extra few hundred calories, then wine is a better choice.

8. Beans instead of rice

If I see beans or lentils anywhere on the menu, I'll often ask if the kitchen can use them instead of one of the faster-digesting starches on my plate. Your waiter may be confused, but he or she will usually do it if you ask.

9. Olive oil and vinegar instead of sugary dressing

At some point in the past twenty years salad dressings started being made with ridiculous amounts of sugar and salt, probably to cover up the completely flavorless vegetables from the industrial food chain. Good old-fashioned olive oil and vinegar make a better choice, and most kitchens have them.

10. Anything instead of American cheese

Have you ever looked at the ingredients in American cheese? Besides water, the first ingredient is usually trans fat. The second is cornstarch. All the way at the bottom it says, "Contains: Milk." Replacing it with real cheddar, gruyère, provolone, or even nothing would be healthier.

LOCKED IN CHAINS

Things start to get ugly when the restaurant selection is no longer up to you. Every now and then, often while visiting family or traveling for work, I find myself in a restaurant, chosen by others, that is just straight-up bad. You know the place: the ingredients are crappy and the portions huge, and sometimes you can smell the industrial oil burning in the back. There's a good chance it is also a chain restaurant. At times like these I go into survival mode.

Although I'm a firm believer that life should be awesome, sometimes it isn't, and we have to make do with what we have. There's no point in complaining and having everyone call you a snob.* Just smile politely, search the menu for the healthiest thing you can find, substitute to your heart's content, eat slowly and mindfully, eat only as much as you need to keep you from starving, and call it a day. The important thing to remember at places like this is that none of the food is going to be good, so you might as well suffer through a flaccid salad or chalky grilled fish and vegetables rather than waste a perfectly good indulgence on something that isn't worth the calories. You can make it up to yourself later.

MENU-SPEAK

Deciphering what is healthy on a menu is not always straightforward. Restaurants have made an art of luring you in with their words and making dishes sound absolutely irresistible, regardless of how they actually taste. Another problem is that dishes that should be healthy, for instance, a Thai chicken salad, are often loaded with secret ingredients (usually extra sugar, salt, and processed oils) that actually cause them

---

* More on this later, but caring about the quality and safety of what you put in your body does not make you a snob. However, judging others for not feeling the same way you do certainly does.

to clock in at way over the number of calories you'd expect (according to the nutrition facts, the Thai chicken salad at California Pizza Kitchen has 1,160 calories). To avoid these traps you need to first learn to decipher menu-speak and then tailor your ordering and special requests to remove the worst offenders.

You already know to avoid foods that are obviously very processed, focus on whole foods, and make sure there is something green on your plate. Once you've gotten that far, the biggest issues are usually sauces and toppings. Sugar, oil, and salt make foods taste better, and when restaurants use low-quality (i.e., bad-tasting) ingredients, they aren't shy about compensating for this by using as many sweet or creamy sauces as possible. Think of these ingredients—the flavor trifecta of sugar, fat, and salt—as makeup for your food. A small amount of the good stuff (e.g., butter or cheese), used tastefully and with restraint, can enhance and beautify a dish. But too much of it is a sign that people are covering up something they don't want you to see.

20 Code Words to Look for on Restaurant Menus

Words to Avoid	Words to Order
glazed	roasted
crispy	baked
melted	broiled
smothered	rubbed
breaded	seared
creamy	grilled
honey-dipped	steamed
crusted	sautéed
gooey	spiced
cheesy	seasoned

How do you know if a restaurant is trying to mask its food with shameless flavor enhancers? Several code words and descriptions can tip you off to this sort of culinary cover-up. Sugar, for example, tends to be sticky, so words like "glaze" and even "sticky" itself are a good sign there is extra sweetener around. Similarly, anything that's "crispy" or "crusted" has likely been covered in a batter made from processed wheat or corn and soaked in oil at high temperatures. Fortunately, there are also words that signify more healthily prepared dishes. "Roasted," "grilled," or "spiced" foods have extra flavor without extra calories.

Sometimes it's hard to find something on a menu that isn't smothered in sugar or dredged in bread crumbs. At this point try to simply find the dish that sounds the best and ask your server to leave off the crispy wontons and bring you a side of spinach instead. Once you know what to look for, making the right call will start to come naturally.

VALUE MEAL

Ultimately, the key to navigating restaurants is deciding where the real value lies. When you know a restaurant isn't particularly special, there's no reason to order the most indulgent thing on the menu. Experiment and figure out what makes healthier food taste better to you (extra avocado?) and choose those options if the circumstances don't warrant a splurge. Even when food is exceptional, remember that you don't need to eat all of it to feel satisfied. Count your indulgences and save them for when they are truly worth it.

THIRTEEN

HOW TO WIN OVER FRIENDS AND INFLUENCE FAMILY

"Families are like fudge: mostly sweet with a few nuts."
—ANONYMOUS

"As a child my family's menu consisted of two choices: take it or leave it."
—BUDDY HACKETT, AMERICAN COMEDIAN

"Language is the means of getting an idea from my brain
into yours without surgery."
—MARK AMIDON

Getting over your own issues with food is one thing, but getting friends and family to support (and hopefully join) you is another story entirely. Everyone knows we should be eating healthier, working out more, and generally making better life decisions. The problem is, once you actually start doing those things, nobody wants to hear about it.

As ridiculous as it sounds, people don't like to know when other people are taking the initiative to do things they know they should be doing themselves but haven't had the discipline to start. If you aren't careful about it, your best efforts can earn you enemies or, worse, lose you friends. No one likes to be reminded of their own failings, and some folks will inevitably view your virtuous behavior as a judgment against their own. This is unfortunate, but it is also normal.

Eating like a foodist does not doom you to being ostracized from your friends and family, however. This chapter will teach you how to lightheartedly deflect your critics, winning them over with charm and tasty, tasty food. We'll also discuss how to gently nudge (but not annoy) those loved ones you hope will adopt some better eating habits for their own sake. This is tricky business for sure, but with an open heart and delicious food, anything is possible.

WORDS WITH FRIENDS

Step one in dealing with the social aspects of eating like a foodist is understanding that criticism almost always stems from a lack of information, personal insecurities, or a combination of both, especially in the realms of food and health. This means that you shouldn't immediately interpret any questioning of your eating habits as a personal attack. Instead, think of them as an invitation to explain your actions and motivations in a friendly, nonthreatening way. Rather than getting defensive or shrinking away in shame, be prepared with a handful of agreeable responses that describe your reasoning, but also make it clear that your actions are in no way a judgment on anyone else's behavior.

The most important tool you have for striking this balance is the language you use to describe your food and habits. In psychology this is known as the *framing effect*. Framing is powerful, because people can have drastically different reactions to exactly the same behavior depending on how they look at it. For instance, if you frame your decision to bring in a salad for lunch as a personal experiment to see if it makes you feel better, your coworkers will be much more sympathetic than if you bring in a salad and self-righteously explain that eating pizza every day isn't healthy. People can relate to wanting to solve personal health issues, but generic statements about what is and isn't right to eat gives the impression that you believe everyone who eats pizza is making a bad life choice. If people believe they are being judged, their natural reaction is to judge you right back. And clearly, you're a jerk.

Whenever possible, avoid framing your choices in a way that implies a value judgment. Steer clear of explanations that emphasize restriction, sacrifice, or self-discipline, since these all imply a negative evaluation of the opposite behavior. Instead, frame your actions in a positive light by highlighting pleasure, enjoyment, and well-being as the motivation behind your actions. You control how you frame your food choices, and the words you use can have a profound impact on how your friends, family, and coworkers respond to them.

The framing effect also works for specific foods. When you frame a food in a positive light by using words that highlight its most delicious attributes rather than its virtuous ones, it can alter the attractiveness of the food as well as how the food is perceived while eaten. This is because taste is subjective, and people actually rate food as tasting better or worse depending on how it is described and presented. Moreover, food that is described as "tasty" is rated as being more satisfying and filling than the same food described as "healthy." The implications of this are huge.

In his book *Marketing Nutrition,* Brian Wansink (the same man who helped us eat less using the mindless margin in his other book, *Mindless Eating*) explores the impact of describing foods in both a positive and negative light. In one experiment, Wansink and his colleagues altered the names of six menu items at a cafeteria at the University of Illinois and observed how well they sold. They also conducted a survey asking patrons to rate the attractiveness, tastiness, and satisfaction (approximate number of calories) of each item. In the control conditions the items had names like "red beans and rice" and "grilled chicken," whereas in the experimental conditions the items were renamed "Traditional Cajun red beans with rice" and "Tender grilled chicken." The

How to Eat Healthy Without Being a Buzzkill

Over the past several years I've used a handful of different tactics to deflect the worst intentions of naysayers. Here are the ones I've found work best.

1. Don't get defensive

The worst thing you can do when some criticizes you for ordering a salad is to get defensive and start preaching your nutritional superiority. I've seen this done, and it doesn't end well. Whatever you do, keep an upbeat tone and maintain perspective. Not everyone understands the importance of their daily food decisions, and it's not your job to educate them.

INSTEAD OF: *"At least I'm not going to have diabetes by the time I'm forty!"*

TRY: *"Actually the salad here is tasty as hell. Have you tried it?"*

2. Use humor

Without getting defensive, you can still jab back a bit, so long as it is clear you're being playful and joking. If someone asks why you aren't eating from the giant tub of stale generic cookies, cracking a joke about how it isn't your vice of choice today can break the ice and get the attention off your healthy decision.

INSTEAD OF: *"Eeeewwwww. Haven't you ever eaten a real cookie?"*

TRY: *"Thanks, but I'm saving my heart attack for the weekend."*

3. Order creatively

No one will make fun of you for making healthier decisions if they don't notice. Ordering a burger and dissecting the meat from the bun is certain to draw attention, but there are plenty of things you can order that won't cause a second glance.

INSTEAD OF: *"Do your meatballs have bread crumbs? Okay, I'll have the spaghetti and meatballs without the sauce and without the spa-*

ghetti, and with extra meatballs. Oh, and a side of steamed broccoli, please."

TRY: "I'll have the steak and spinach salad with a glass of your best California cab, please. And can I get some blue cheese with that as well?"

4. Use happy honesty

It's hard for people to say bad things about you if you come across as happy and at peace with your decisions, especially if it's clear you aren't being motivated by your ego.

INSTEAD OF: "I'm choosing salad, because I'd really like to lose ten pounds this year, so I don't end up looking like you."

TRY: "I'm just trying to eat a little healthier these days to see how it makes me feel."

5. Use harmless lies

Honesty is always the best policy, except when you're trying to get your jerk coworkers off your back so you can enjoy your lunch.

INSTEAD OF: "I'm eating a smaller lunch today, so I can hit the gym later."

TRY: "I had a really big breakfast. I'm just not that hungry."

6. Share alike

If you know in advance you're going to be bringing your own food, you have the advantage of having a meal that looks, smells, and tastes much better than anything your friends will find at the corner sandwich shop. Show off your amazing new flavors by bringing enough of something delicious to share.

INSTEAD OF: "Yuck, I can't believe you're eating that disgusting excuse for a calzone."

TRY: "Have you tried the mandarins from the farmers market this season? They're freaking amazing! Here, I have an extra one."

7. Accept and nibble

Friends can be very crafty and sometimes try and force you into eating unhealthy food by offering it to you point-blank. Cheap office birthday cakes are particularly offensive. Politely turning down the objectionable substance is one strategy, but it can easily backfire. Just gratefully accept the food and pretend to eat it.

INSTEAD OF: *"Just a small piece for me, please."*

TRY: *"Mmm . . . thanks."*

Take one bite, keep smiling, and continue the conversation while leaving the food nonchalantly on the table. When everyone else is finishing up, subtly drop it in the trash without making a fuss (trust me, nothing is going to waste). By that time, no one will care what you're doing. If someone does say something, just blame it on how big of a piece you were served.

8. Don't offer unsolicited advice

No matter how tempting it is, don't be the reverse jerk. Only offer nutrition advice to friends if they explicitly ask you for it; otherwise keep your trap shut. The best thing you can do to help your friends is show them what good healthy food looks and tastes like by setting a good example; then let them watch for themselves as you lose weight and get in shape.

INSTEAD OF: *"You know, that Lean Cuisine isn't going to help you get rid of those thunder thighs."*

TRY: *"Yes, I have lost weight! Thanks for noticing! Yeah, I've been reading this book called* Foodist. *It's great. You should check it out."*

descriptive titles increased sales by 27 percent, and the diners rated these items as more appealing, tastier, and higher in calories (remember they were exactly the same foods).[1] According to Wansink, "Descriptive labels influenced nearly every aspect of the eating experience."[2]

You can make healthy food sound (and therefore taste) more delicious by describing it using words that evoke a geographical location, tradition, nostalgia, or vivid sensory images. This should be easy for a foodist, since real food is innately rich in these attributes. Real food is "farm fresh," "seasonal," "ripe," "hand-picked," "crisp," "succulent," and "juicy," and you can use all these words to your advantage. Similarly, if you've taken care to prepare an ingredient in a special way, you can use language that emphasizes your cooking method. Did you make those ravioli by hand or slow roast that pork shoulder? Play it up. Remember that you aren't just serving delicious healthy food—you have to sell it. If you're excited about something you found at the farmers market, explain why. Tell stories about where the food comes from or the interesting new recipe you found.

Getting your friends and family excited about healthy food begins long before anyone sits down at the table. Every time someone asks you what's for dinner, you have the opportunity to make your food taste better and be more satisfying. Think of it as seasoning with words. Be careful, however, to not oversell your wares. If you just talk the talk, but don't walk the walk, people may lose confidence in what you say and be inclined to stop eating healthy food entirely. For your own sake and the sake of others, always strive to serve food you really enjoy that looks, smells, and tastes amazing.

Interestingly, Wansink suggests that the reason descriptive language changes our experience of food so dramatically is that it encourages mindful eating. "Part of what descriptive labeling allows consumers to do is to concentrate more on their feelings and on the taste of the foods," says Wansink.[3] People in his cafeteria experiment who ate foods with descriptive labels focused the vast majority, 84 percent, of their comments on describing the sensory elements of food, such as its taste or texture, whereas those who ate the foods with regular labels only mentioned sensory attributes in 42 percent of their comments; the latter group tended to highlight the functional characteristics of the foods, such as the price.

50 Mouthwatering Words to Describe Real Food

farm fresh	poached	dry-aged	slow-roasted
fall	summer	whisked	juicy
chilled	baby	rubbed	crisp
savory	imported	rich	braised
roasted	bacon-laced	seasonal	steeped
organic	grilled	tender	handmade
winter	tasty	scented	marinated
warm	heirloom	slow-cooked	spring
smoky	fresh	hand-picked	succulent
aromatic	seared	late-season	sautéed
sweet	drizzled	colorful	hand-tossed
local	tangy	tossed	crusted
toasted	young		

Once again we see that eating mindfully helps us enjoy food more, and eat less of it. This is especially useful when you're trying to help people enjoy healthier foods, which are often viewed as being less satisfying and filling than what are perceived as normal or fattening foods. Describing a food as healthy* gives it a "health halo," which Wansink has demonstrated causes people to underestimate the number of calories in the food and overeat more fattening foods later (since they've been so virtuous and earned a treat).[4] Amazingly, people tend to eat even more calories when they perceive a food as healthy than they do if they believe a food is fattening. And of course they don't realize it, causing them to miscalculate their intake by hundreds of calories. Using descriptive language to enhance the appeal of healthy foods actu-

---

* Or "low-fat," "low-carb," "trans fat–free," "low glycemic index," "high-fiber," "gluten-free," "containing soy," or any other health buzzword.

ally shifts them in your mind away from "healthy and unsatisfying" to "delicious and filling," thereby reducing your risk of unintentionally overeating.

The power of language to impact your food experience can work in the opposite direction as well. For average individuals who are not particularly health-conscious, any mention of an ingredient that is considered healthy (and therefore bad tasting) is likely to negatively impact their enjoyment of the food. In another set of experiments, Wansink examined this effect by offering people nutrition bars with different labels. For one group the labels claimed that the bar contained "10 grams of soy protein," and for another the label said "10 grams of protein." Inside the package the bars were identical, and neither batch contained soy. The people who were given the bars without the term "soy" on the labeling generally liked them and had positive comments about the taste and texture, but those who had been given the bars they believed contained soy rated them far less favorably.[5] In the experiment people had preconceived notions about the taste of soy, and this bias shaded their experience of the food. "People will taste what they expect to taste, and it's important to not negatively bias expectations," says Wansink.[6]

There is a small percentage of the population, those who call themselves "health-conscious," who do not exhibit a negative bias when a food is described as healthy. But it is important to remember that for most people healthy food isn't very appealing, so it's best not to mention it. Instead, focus on the tasty attributes of your food, and maybe your eaters will forget that your roasted cauliflower is actually good for them.

"BROCCOLI HELPS ME GROW"

To the dismay of many, child psychology is not the same as adult psychology, and getting kids to eat vegetables requires a slightly different approach. Though I don't have children myself, I have spoken with countless people about their kids' eating habits, and those who have successfully integrated whole, unprocessed foods into their families' healthstyle share many similarities.

I was never a picky eater as a child. Sure, I would occasionally hide an asparagus spear under my excess mashed potatoes, but for the most part I ate my broccoli, peas, and carrots without complaint. I also ate spicy salsa, sushi, mustard, onions, and chicken liver paté. When I asked my dad why he believed this was the case, he echoed what I've heard from parents all over the world. I ate what was offered, because he and my mother never expected me do to anything else; I was never given the option of special meals, so it never occurred to me to ask for them. Accommodating picky eaters with special foods or meals reinforces the message that rejecting foods is acceptable behavior and discourages adventurous eating.

One of the biggest factors impacting children's acceptance of food is the behavior and eating preferences of their parents.[7] I was five years old the first time my parents took me and my younger brother, Dana, to a sushi restaurant. They didn't tell us we were going to eat raw fish and seaweed, just that we were going to try a Japanese restaurant they loved. When we got there, the waitstaff were all wearing beautiful kimonos, and we were escorted to a low table where there were mats to sit on the floor. Dana and I didn't think this was scary; we thought it was the coolest thing ever. Our waiter explained to us that it was traditional to eat Japanese food with chopsticks and rigged us each up with a pair that were banded together with some paper and a rubber band at the end so they worked like tweezers. I was willing to eat anything, so long as I was allowed to use these awesome new chopsticks.

My parents ordered everything they normally would, including sushi rolls, tempura shrimp and vegetables, and also some beef teriyaki and fried chicken, which they knew we would like. Still, they offered us everything and suggested we try it if we were interested. We did focus most of our attention on the chicken and beef that first day, but loved the crispy tempura vegetables and even a few bites of sushi roll. We didn't even think it was weird. I found out later that sushi was made from raw fish and seaweed, but by then it was already one of my favorite foods and I didn't really care.

Making food fun is one of the most effective ways to convince kids to try new things. Recent research from Wansink and others shows that children actually prefer more diverse and colorful plates than adults.[8] They also prefer it when the foods are arranged more sparsely rather than clumped together in the center of the plate. If the food is made into shapes or patterns on the plate, even better. Some parents have reported success with making a game of eating, such as telling children that they are dinosaurs and that broccoli florets are tiny trees that need to be eaten. Children also respond better to the idea of eating foods that "help them grow" than to commandments followed by "Because I said so."

Research consistently shows that kids who initially reject a food must be exposed to it repeatedly (at least eight to ten attempts) for it to be accepted. Many parents have had success with the "one bite rule": a child must try at least one solid bite of each food every time it is presented. Some research has shown that rewarding this behavior with things like stickers helps children be more adventurous and eventually leads to better long-term acceptance of the food.[9] In contrast, putting negative pressure on a child to eat foods can backfire by turning mealtime into an all-around unpleasant experience, which can actually increase picky-eating tendencies.[10]

When reintroducing foods, try different preparations and cooking methods to make the food more appealing. Surrounding a rejected food with flavors the child normally likes, like cheese or bacon, can be especially effective. This was a favorite trick in my own household when I was growing up. "If I'd melted cheese on it, you guys would have eaten shoe leather," my dad told me when I asked him why he thought we always ate our vegetables. I've spoken to other parents who swear that garlic, salt, and pepper is a combination enticing enough to get their kids to eat almost anything. The important thing is to get children accustomed to eating a diverse assortment of fresh vegetables and fruits. As long as the garnishes are made from real ingredients, a few extra calories that help them enjoy the experience is perfectly fine.

I'm less a fan of hiding healthy ingredients in foods, like grinding up spinach and putting it into brownies. The goal should be to get children to enjoy real food, and hiding vegetables only sends the message that they aren't important enough to eat for their own sake. I would only suggest this as a last resort for extremely picky children.

Children are more invested in a meal if they help with its preparation. Take your kids with you to the farmers market and introduce them to the farmers who grow their food. Better yet, start a garden and teach them how to plant and harvest their own. Invite them into the kitchen and let them help clean carrots, snap beans, mix the salad dressing, and set the table. Letting your children participate in the process gives them a sense of pride, and they feel a deeper connection with their food, making them much more excited about eating it.

All children are different, and clearly some will be more difficult to cajole than others. As a parent, you can just do your best with the tools you have. Create as many positive food experiences as you can and never complain about food-related chores such as shopping, cooking, or cleaning the kitchen. Set a good example and keep trying. Picky eating is a state of mind, but it doesn't need to be a way of life.

FOODIST AND FAMILY

One of the toughest situations a foodist can encounter is seeing loved ones suffer as a result of their eating habits. Traditional whole foods have been out of fashion for so long that many of our parents and sometimes even our grandparents are completely unaware of the negative health effects caused by the foods they grew up loving. As they age, however, these habits start to take their toll, and we must watch as their health deteriorates. A medical emergency that brings them face-to-face with reality is sometimes what it takes for them to make changes. Other times even that isn't enough.

Unfortunately, changing the habits of another person is even more difficult than changing your own. Stubbornness, pride, and ignorance can prevent people from even listening to advice that could save their lives, and for whatever reason age tends to compound these particular traits. Pushing a message that people don't want to hear can cause them to dig in and fight even harder to preserve their way of life, straining and potentially destroying your relationship with them. When dealing with someone like this, it's first essential to accept the fact that there may be nothing you can do for him or her. No matter how badly you may desire to help, a person has to want to change and cannot be forced.

But still, change can happen. Despite my close relationship with my father and his enthusiasm about my career path, I didn't expect him to ever alter the way he ate. My dad had suffered from depression since I was in high school, and his outlook got even worse after my mother passed away in a car accident in 2003. Like most people he had developed the habit of eating processed and fast foods starting in the early 1990s, and as his depression grew deeper, the effort he put into feeding and taking care of himself waned.

"In general, I did not want to continue living and didn't think I would. With all the health problems I was having, and especially after your mom died—that was a really hard thing for me to deal with— and I thought it would be better if I was gone too," he told me.

After a series of serious medical emergencies that nearly took his life on three occasions, I had nearly given up hoping for a turnaround, even though he was only in his fifties. But I continued to love him and share my passion for seasonal food whenever possible.

"You were so understanding, you never put any pressure on me or tried to convince me to change, but you always gave me hope that things would get better, things would be better," he recalled.

From my perspective he had gone through enough and didn't need me or anyone else telling him how to live out his life. If he didn't want to live, I didn't want to bug him about his blood pressure or eating habits. I just wanted to have as many happy and positive times with him as possible until whatever happened happened, and the last thing I wanted was to strain our relationship unnecessarily. I know my dad, and he is not one to do anything just because someone else, even me, thinks he should. Still my excitement about food and health was genuine, and I knew he had always been a fan of a good meal, so I continued to share what I was learning.

My cooking was the first thing that caught his attention. I made a point whenever visiting home in southern California to stop by the San Francisco farmers market before getting on the plane and bringing back something delicious. On one summer trip I brought home a small bag of padrón peppers, some good olive oil, and a crusty baguette. Padróns are small green peppers that are a common *tapas* dish in Spain and a seasonal delicacy for foodists in San Francisco. They are incredibly simple to prepare. All you have to do is heat some olive oil in a cast-iron pan and cook the peppers over medium heat until they blister and just start to brown. When they're done, sprinkle them with some coarse sea salt and eat them with your fingers. Padróns have a deep pepper flavor, but are not usually spicy—except when they are. One out of every ten peppers is incredibly hot, so eating a bowl is a bit like playing Russian roulette with your tongue.

My dad has always been a fan of spicy foods, and I knew that padróns would be right up his alley. At his house I cooked them with a little more olive oil than usual, because it becomes infused with the oil from the peppers and tastes delicious. We used the bread to sop up the extra pepper oil and cool our mouths when we got burned on the spicy ones. My dad loved every bit of it and quietly started paying more attention whenever I mentioned food.

His next great epiphany was beets. All his life he had hated beets, and consequently I had never eaten them as a child. The first couple of times I tried them, even at nice restaurants, beets tasted a little off to me. Something about their flavor reminded me of dirt, and I could never get past that to enjoy their earthy sweetness. But I continued to sample them when they were available, hoping one day something would click. That day came one sunny afternoon at the house of a friend who was hosting a dinner party. We were having Dungeness crab for dinner, which I was totally excited about, but the main course was a long way off, so she put out a huge pile of roasted beets sprinkled with chèvre cheese and fresh mint as an appetizer.

I was starving, so I started reluctantly picking at the giant pile with my fingers, since I didn't want to scoop myself a serving of food I didn't expect to like. I popped the first bite in my mouth and, yeah, it still tasted like beets. But I was hungry, so I tried another, this time with a good portion of mint and cheese on it. After a few chews, it hit me. "Whoa, this is good," I said to myself. Something about the fresh-tasting mint and the creamy cheese balanced the earthy flavor of the beets and transformed them into something I could appreciate. I proceeded to put a hefty dent in the beet mountain, leaving bright pink stains all over my fingers. Beets had finally made it onto my beloved vegetables list, and I started making my own version of the recipe at home.

Proud of my recent conversion, I told my dad about my beet discovery during our next phone conversation. He replied skeptically, saying that he hated beets and always had. But I knew I was onto something and decided to include the recipe in our next Thanksgiving dinner, just so he could try it for himself. I made plenty of other dishes as well, just in case he really didn't like the beets, but I followed my friend's lead and set them out earlier than the rest of the food as an appetizer, knowing that someone with a hungry tummy couldn't resist trying a bite. It worked.

Beating Beet Aversions

If my dad can learn to like beets at the age of fifty-five, anyone can. This is the recipe that convinced him (and me a year earlier) that the humble beet can be as delicious and elegant as any exotic vegetable.

This is the perfect dish for the beet skeptic and beet lover alike, and it hardly requires any cooking skills. If you are still worried you will not like the flavor of beets, look for the milder and less messy golden or pink- and white-striped cioggia beets. Whenever possible I like to use a few different colors to mix it up, but if all you have are the common red garden beets they work beautifully on their own.

To begin you must eliminate all thoughts of substituting canned beets for fresh. Fresh roasted beets have a rich, sweet, earthy flavor that is completely unlike that of the flaccid purple slivers that come in a can. You will also need fresh mint leaves. Most grocery stores carry them; ask if you can't find them. Chèvre is a soft goat cheese that a close friend of mine describes as "like cream cheese only better." A little bit goes a very long way, so I always buy the smallest amount possible (it usually costs around $3).

Be careful not to add the cheese directly to hot beets or it will melt and form an unattractive pink slime. It still tastes good, but it's better to avoid this problem by cooling the beets beforehand. An hour in the refrigerator works well, but if you are in a hurry you can get away with ten to fifteen minutes in the freezer. This dish is very easy to scale for large batches, making it ideal for parties and potlucks.

Roasted Beets with Fresh Mint and Chèvre
SERVES 2 TO 3

1 bunch of beets (3 large), any variety
1 to 2 tablespoons olive oil
½ cup fresh mint leaves, loosely packed
¼ ounce chèvre
Sea salt or kosher salt

Preheat the oven to 375°F. If the leaves are still on the beets, twist them off, leaving enough stem to use as a handle for peeling. (If the beet greens are still fresh and springy, I recommend cleaning them and cooking them up with some onions and garlic—sauté them like spinach. Beet greens are so full of potassium that they taste naturally salty, so be careful with your seasoning, because they are easy to oversalt.)

Peel the beets using a vegetable peeler and chop them evenly into ¾- to 1-inch cubes. Keep in mind that the larger the pieces, the longer they will take to cook. Discard stems.

Add the olive oil to the beets and toss to coat. Sprinkle the beets with salt and place in a single layer in a large Pyrex baking pan. Place the pan in the oven on the middle rack and roast until the beets are tender and have a glazed-like appearance, stirring every 8 to 10 minutes. Roasting takes approximately 35 minutes.

When the beets are finished roasting, transfer them to a large bowl, cover with plastic wrap, and place in the refrigerator. Chill for at least 30 minutes, but 45 to 60 minutes is preferable. Five minutes before the beets are done chilling, stack the mint leaves on top of each other and chiffonade them by rolling them lengthwise like a cigarette and slicing them into thin ribbons. For very large leaves I like to cut the ribbons in half once by making a single cut through the middle of the pile along the vein of the leaves. Discard the stems.

Using a fork, crumble a small amount of the chèvre into a small bowl or plate and set it aside. When the beets are ready, sprinkle the mint onto the beets and stir, reserving a few ribbons for garnish. Adjust salt to taste. Transfer the minted beets to a serving bowl and sprinkle with the chèvre and remaining mint. Serve immediately.

"When you made those beets I was like, 'Wow, this is so unbelievable! So different from what I remember,'" he recalled.

I was stoked, and my dad became a believer. At almost sixty years old, he developed a new appreciation for vegetables and real food (turns out the beets he grew up eating were always from a can), even the ones he thought he didn't like.

"It made eating and preparing healthy food much more fascinating," he explained. "It became exciting to me to see what the possibilities are."

The beets weren't enough to change my dad's habits, but he was starting to make the connection between good food and good health. More important, he was now convinced that vegetables and other healthy foods could taste amazing and that eating them would not be a sacrifice. He also began paying more attention to me and the things I would say and share on Facebook about the connections between food and wellness.

Though he still didn't care much about his own life or health, he was growing weary of feeling sick and drained all the time, and it was becoming obvious to him that his health (and possibly his diet) was the reason. After living for decades on processed foods, my dad had developed prediabetes and his blood sugar swings were having a terrible impact on his mood and energy levels. He also had dangerously high blood pressure, and in 2006 a mild stroke left him with a speech impediment that deeply troubled and embarrassed him. Worse, the stroke made it nearly impossible for him to play his guitar, the only passion he had left in his life. Though he was able to recover his speech and dexterity after a couple of months, this experience scared him enough to at least start taking medication for his condition and paying more attention to his diet. He may not have cared then if he lived or died, but he knew he didn't want to live without his music.

Because he's a good father, my dad had always done his best to keep up with my work ever since I started writing in 2007. He's seen almost all my rants against processed food and praise for seasonal vegetables, pastured eggs, and wild fish, and nothing had ever convinced him to change the way he eats. Then one day in late July 2011, I got a phone call with the words I never expected to hear.

A few weeks earlier I had released a video on Summer Tomato about salt, explaining how it affects your health and what you need to understand to make smart food decisions. My basic argument was that salt itself is not bad for you. In fact, it is necessary to have some sodium in your diet. Moreover, salt makes food taste better, and I encourage everyone to sprinkle some on their vegetables if it helps them eat more of them. There are three reasons salt is a problem for most Western societies. The first is that we eat way too much of it, which can lead to hypertension. However, a whopping 75 percent of the sodium we eat comes from processed foods.[11] Relatively speaking, the salt you add to your own home-cooked food is insignificant.

The second issue is that sodium intake must be balanced by sufficient potassium intake, which comes mainly from vegetables. That is, the more vegetables you eat, the less dietary sodium matters. Most people don't eat enough vegetables, so eating a lot of sodium poses a bigger risk for developing high blood pressure than it would in the context of a healthier diet.[12] Third, a high intake of fructose, a common ingredient in processed foods, exacerbates the effects of sodium in the diet.[13] This means that the same amount of salt in your food is more dangerous if there is a lot of fructose around as well. All three of these points lead to the simple conclusion that too many processed foods and too few vegetables are the real causes of hypertension, not the little white shaker sitting on your kitchen table.

On that random day in July my dad called to tell me that he watched this video, and something about it struck a chord. I remember his words so vividly I can still hear him saying them in my head.

"I watched that video you made about salt, and it was really great," he began.

"Thanks, Dad," I replied.

"Yeah, I was watching it, and you made me realize that salt is already inside the processed foods," he explained.

"That's right," I answered, almost chuckling at his excitement about this simple revelation. My brain instantly cued the scene from the movie *Zoolander* in which Hansel realizes that files are kept *in the computer* and then throws the machine off a balcony, so he could open it up and find them.

"Well, since the salt is already in there, I stopped eating them," he continued.

"What?" I wasn't sure I'd heard him right.

"I stopped eating the processed foods a couple weeks ago. But I needed something else to eat, and I remembered you always saying I'm supposed to eat vegetables, so I went to the store and bought all of them," he went on.

"What? What did you buy?" I asked, starting to realize the meaning of his words. Maybe he did throw his processed foods off the balcony.

"I bought all the vegetables. They weren't very well labeled, so I wasn't sure exactly what I was getting. But I think I got some kale and some chard. And I got some peppers, onions, mushrooms, and all sorts of other weird shit. I took it home and cut it all up—it took an hour there was so much of it—and I made three huge batches of stir-fry. It was beautiful, and so colorful, so I call it my Rainbow Stir-Fry. And it was delicious! I take it to work and eat it every day for breakfast and lunch. I also sauté some fish or turkey meat and eat that. After eating that all day, I'm not usually hungry for dinner."

Laughing again, this time in disbelief, I asked, "So you've been eating nothing but vegetables, fish, and turkey for two weeks?"

"Yeah, and I love it! And I've had to poke two new holes in my belt. I think I'll need to get new pants soon."

To say this was hard to believe is beyond an understatement. Seemingly overnight, my dad, who had nearly given up on his own life, had completely overhauled his eating habits and loved everything about it. At the time I didn't let myself dwell too long on what this could mean. It was still too new, and too unbelievable. But deep down I knew what was at stake if he was serious: it meant he might make it. It meant he might be around to meet his future grandkids, my future children.

As I hoped, my dad's change was real and permanent. In just two months he was down twenty-five pounds. I know this because he was so impressed by his own transformation that he went and bought himself a scale to track his progress. It wasn't out of vanity—the man doesn't have a full-length mirror in his entire house—but out of curiosity. He wanted to have something tangible to look at and know that what he was doing was making a difference.

"In the beginning I didn't know I was losing weight because I didn't weigh myself, but I kept having to put new holes in my belt, and one day there were so many folds in my pants. I wore a size 36, so I tried a 34, and goddamn those were too big! I couldn't believe I was a size 32—I was so proud of myself."

Shortly after that he developed an uncontrollable urge to start exercising.

"It only took about two to three weeks of me eating like that every day to feel a complete difference in my body, in the way I felt. It all starts adding together, it has an effect on your whole life," he explained. "The exercise came along when the weight started melting off. It was just dropping off me. And I felt like I wanted to stretch and move again. I didn't want to feel weak anymore," he said.

For over five years he had been using a cane to walk. His knee had been severely weakened from a staph infection, which required surgery that left a massive amount of scar tissue. But when he started losing weight, it was easier for him to move around, and he started using the cane less and less. He started taking the stairs instead of the elevator at work, spent more time walking with his dogs, and bought some used exercise equipment for his house—some dumbbells and an ab roller wheel. Over a year later he is down fifty pounds and doesn't use a cane at all.

"Now I do a hundred ab rolls every day,"* he told me. "I remember when I hit eighty the first time I couldn't believe it. It's really good because when things don't go well at work one day, or I have problems with the dogs, I know I did my hundred rolls. I have at least that one thing I'm proud of. It's a lifestyle that I find very delightful," he gushed.

As his eating habits and body transformed, so did his outlook on life.

"I thought, 'Well shit, if I'm going to live and see my kids grow up, I don't want to be in a wheelchair. I better be fit enough to do stuff on this planet,'" he explained.

When I asked him what he thought led to his change, he had a hard time putting his finger on it.

He said, "For me it took having the wake-up call of the health issue. Then somewhere in me I decided I really didn't want to die. I don't know exactly when it was, but it was definitely associated with you. I always felt better after speaking to you. It wasn't for me or because of me, but your belief that things could be better."

My dad's healthstyle has evolved since he first started on his journey. Eventually he became tired of eating his Rainbow Stir-Fry day in and day out.

"At first," he explained, "it was a bit like cooking dinner and making a piece of art you could eat. Then after about six months it started being too much of a hassle and started getting old. But that didn't mean I went back to my old habits."

He now shops and cooks more frequently, making smaller batches of vegetables and fish that he can whip up quickly in the morning before work. "I mix it up with different sauces, Chinese or Turkish, and I rotate and shop at different places for my vegetables. I found a little

---

*If you've ever tried these you know how hard they are. I can only do about thirty, and then I'm sore for days.

produce place by my house now that has better vegetables than my grocery store. I never get tired of this stuff."

Though he knows his dishes and strategies will continue to change as he gets better at cooking and learns to use new vegetables, he isn't worried about slipping back into his former habits.

"I've gone long enough now that I know in my heart that I'll never go back to my old way of eating, because I don't find any joy in it. I still go get sushi or Mexican food occasionally, but I don't want to do it every day. I'm happy and comfortable with how I'm doing it now."

My video on salt was clearly a catalyst for my dad's turnaround, but it would have been impossible for it to have had the impact it did without the years of education and encouragement from me that came before it. Just as important is that he was able to make the adjustments at his own pace, without pressure from anyone to do it a certain way.

"I was able to read on Summer Tomato without interacting with you all the time, and see the reasons for doing all this stuff. Then I had the opportunity and knowledge, which I got because of you, and I stumbled my way through it until I got my own style. Once I made up my mind, I'm pretty hard to keep down. I went whole hog," he explained.

I asked him if he had any advice for people in the same situation that I was in, wanting to help a loved one make healthier choices.

"As long as they can be patient and present things in a way that's easy to understand. Let your family see how you eat, read a little, and get some inspiration. Everyone has to find their own path, what works for them," he advised.

As for my dad, he's just happy it clicked for him when it did.

"I'm feeling better now than I have in a really, really long time. I'm very confident about the future," he said.

"So am I." I smiled.

FOURTEEN

ON FOOD
AND VALUES

"Food for thought is no substitute for the real thing."
—WALT KELLY

"I arise in the morning torn between a desire to improve the world and a desire to enjoy the world. This makes it hard to plan the day."
—E. B. WHITE

"Reading without reflecting is like eating without digesting."
—EDMUND BURKE

What you choose to eat can have a profound impact on your quality of life. But as we've seen, even the best choices are only as powerful as your ability to implement them consistently, something that is not always as straightforward as we'd like it to be. So far I've outlined dozens of tips and tricks you can use to make healthy choices easier, but I've neglected to mention the single most powerful motivator for following through on your goals: conviction.

Ever wonder why Muslims can endure strict fasting for a month during Ramadan, but you can't avoid eating that second doughnut during your weekly strategy meeting? People whose food choices are driven by their personal values are not lured by temptation, because they believe their actions have meaning above and beyond their own hedonistic desires. Vegetarians, vegans, and people of faith who follow strict dietary rules believe, with conviction, that making choices that are consistent with their values is more important than whatever inconveniences come from them. As a result, their choices are clear and they have little trouble following through on them.

We all have a set of personal values that we use to define our relationship with the rest of the world and guide our behavior. Unfortunately, there is so little transparency in our modern food chain that we rarely see how our eating habits align with those values. Almost everyone can find reasons to transcend their personal health goals and care more about their food choices, however. By digging a little deeper and further educating ourselves about where our food comes from and how it is produced, we can start to see what we eat as more than something that makes us fat or skinny, healthy or unhealthy. We learn that our food choices have a powerful impact on the world and help define our community and our character. Whether we connect what we eat with food safety, environmental sustainability, religious beliefs, national security, local food economies, culinary artistry, or simple enjoyment, embracing a broader philosophy about the way we eat helps make our food choices more clear, easier to maintain, and ultimately more rewarding.

REMEMBER THE ELEPHANT

Research shows that value-based motivators are more effective for changing people's behavior than health-based ones. In 2010, scientists at Stanford published a study comparing the eating habits of students in four different food-related upper-division biology courses. Three of the courses focused on health, emphasizing the impact of dietary choices on health outcomes, while the experimental "Food and Society" class focused on food-related social issues, but not health. At the end of the semester, only the students in the Food and Society class showed a marked increase in the amount of vegetables and fruits consumed and a decrease in less healthy foods. Ironically, the students in the health courses showed a significant decrease in vegetable consumption over the course of the study. The students in the Food and Society course also reported feeling more strongly about the importance of the environment, animal rights, and a healthful diet, indicating that their new beliefs may have influenced their behavior.[1]

We've already discussed how trying to use willpower day in and day out in order to eat better, exercise more, and lose weight is ineffective. This is largely because the goals of health and weight loss are too abstract and distant to substantially sway your immediate, hedonistic desires. The elephant in your brain is too lazy, and the rider trying to guide it is too weak. However, your elephant will respond to loftier, value-based goals, and these can be some of your most powerful sources of motivation. By educating yourself more on the issues surrounding food, you can fuel your elephant's determination to take the high road and keep the noble course. You might even lose some weight in the process.

FOOD IS NONDENOMINATIONAL

One of the best things about the food movement is that, regardless of your political or spiritual leanings, you can almost certainly find something to get excited about. Food is a relatively nondenominational topic that supports values that range across the political spectrum. Love furry animals and considering going vegetarian? Read up on industrial meat production and the differences between it and humane, sustainable farming. Farmer Joel Salatin's excellent book *Folks, This Ain't Normal* is a great place to start.[2] Worried your family may be exposed to food-safety hazards like those half billion *Salmonella*-tainted eggs recalled in

2010? Learn about the problems with having a centralized food system dominated by industrial food and how supporting smaller, regional farmers can help diversify and strengthen our resources. Books like *Poisoned*, by Jeff Benedict, can help you get the ball rolling.[3]

Choosing foods from smaller, local farms supports regional economies, bolsters small business, and creates more competition, ideals that strongly align with traditional conservative values. Industrial farmers also receive massive government subsidies to overproduce commodity crops like corn, wheat, soybeans, and rice, a practice that is directly responsible for the market flood of cheap junk food. If you don't like the idea of your tax dollars going to fuel this kind of corporate welfare, read up on the Farm Bill and how voting with your fork can impact government policy. For a more liberal perspective, dig into the vast amounts of literature on how agriculture and food production are as bad (or worse) for our environment than even the transportation industry, and how biodynamic and sustainable agriculture practices can reverse this devastating trend. Read books like Barry Estabrook's *Tomatoland* to get a glimpse of the atrocious living and working conditions of industrial farm workers, which have been likened to modern-day slavery.[4] You'll also learn that the (lack of) taste of industrially grown produce isn't simply collateral damage caused by modern agriculture, but that powerful farming interests intentionally suppress the production of tastier tomato varieties in favor of cheaper production and transport.

Politics aside, all of us should be concerned about the proliferation of "superbugs" such as MRSA, new strains of bacteria that are resistant to multiple kinds of antibiotics. Antibiotic drugs are arguably the most important tools we have in containing disease and infection, and as they become less effective, the potential damage to human life and society is immeasurable. About 80 percent of the antibiotics used in the United States go to livestock, most of which is added to their feed and water to promote growth while enabling them to be raised in high-density conditions. Overuse of drugs in this capacity creates selective evolutionary pressure for the development of antibiotic resistance, which has been shown to be directly responsible for the emergence of human strains of superbugs.[5] Antibiotic resistance on farms also increases the risk of deadly food poisoning outbreaks that may be resistant to traditional drugs. Though the FDA is taking steps to limit the use of antibiotics in livestock production, choosing organic and pasture-raised meat products supports responsible farming practices and limits your risk of exposure to antibiotic-resistant *E. coli*.

At a more personal level, cooking and eating real food is fundamental to our most basic human needs and desires, and this gives it tremendous value in its own right. As the late food writer M. F. K. Fisher says in the foreword to *The Art of Eating*, "It seems to me that our three basic needs, for food and security and love, are so mixed and mingled and entwined that we cannot straightly think of one without the others."[6] Although better health for yourself and your family is certainly an important reason for paying more attention to the foods you eat together, the value it brings to your home extends far beyond your BMI and cholesterol levels. Cooking and eating together with family and friends strengthens our relationships with the people who matter most to us. Meals are a time for sharing, learning, and laughing, and as we move away from real food toward processed, manufactured products we lose much of the closeness that cooking and eating together creates. Embracing a tradition of food and cooking serves to build lifelong memories and enrich the time you spend with those you love.

Focusing on food builds ties beyond the family as well. There is something innately comforting about knowing the people who grow (not manufacture) your food. People who care about what they produce delight in sharing their passion. Simply asking a farmer or butcher "What's good today?" will lead to tales about the farm, the weather, and the intricacies of seed selection and pest control. Those stories bind you to your food, your farmer, and your community. If you've spent most of your life without these things, as the majority of us have, they may not seem very important. But historically these relationships are the backbone of our culture and the root of our identity, and restoring them is an important step in healing our bodies and food system.

These community relationships are also more powerful than you might expect in helping you achieve your healthstyle goals. When I think about how hard these farmers work to grow their beautiful produce and trek it to market before the sun comes up every Saturday, part of me can't help but feel obliged to support them in any way I can. What that means is I'm willing to pay more for a peach if I know it's the best one at the market, I'll try a new vegetable because I trust my farmer's dedication to delicious food, and I'll haul myself out of bed on a cold, rainy Saturday just to support the farmers and let them know I'm more than just a fair-weather shopper. In other words, I eat better because I care about them. Although building these deeper relationships isn't necessary for eating well, they give more meaning to the food decisions you make and provide the sort of subtle psychological rewards that strengthen habits and make it easier to fulfill your goals.

Food is also a gateway into new cultures. Traditional cuisines reflect the climate, resources, values, and spirit of different communities around the world. One of my favorite things to do before visiting another country is to buy a cookbook of the area's traditional cuisine and familiarize myself with a few of the signature ingredients and dishes. I do this so that when I get there, I know what to order and can appreciate the cuisine and culture at a deeper level than I could have by ordering at random (though this can be fun too). Having the cookbook also gives me a way to transport myself back there whenever memories and nostalgia get the better of me. I consider it a bonus that traditional cultures are based on real food and are therefore (mostly) good for me.

The topics I've outlined here are just the tip of the iceberg for issues that show us how food contributes to more than just the perkiness of our backsides. Start down the rabbit hole and you may come out a different person, and this is probably a good thing. Understanding the world better makes us more responsible citizens, and if it helps you develop values that trickle onto your dinner plate, it's a double win. Your healthstyle will practically upgrade itself.

If you still aren't quite sure where to start, try renting a copy of the documentary *Food, Inc.* It's entertaining and educational and does a good job of covering some of the most pressing food issues. My only recommendation would be to not have a plate of industrial food in front of you when you turn it on. I saw the film when it was first released at a local theater, and the girl eating a hotdog in the seat next to me nearly lost her cookies when she saw what goes into making industrial meat. The film isn't gory, but it will certainly make you wonder where your dinner has been before it found its way to your plate. If, like me, you're more of a book person, Michael Pollan's *The Omnivore's Dilemma* is one of the most well-written and educational books on modern food I've ever encountered.[7]

FOODIST OR ELITIST?

But isn't all this talk about fancy food and small farms just elitist San Francisco drivel? Isn't organic produce a luxury only the upper middle class can indulge in, like private schools and hybrid cars? The food movement has been attacked from every side, but the accusation of elitism is the one that tends to stick. It's easy to understand why. At the grocery store organic food certainly sports a higher price tag than conventional food, and not everyone has access to farmers markets year-round. Cooking takes time, as does educating yourself about global food-supply issues. These are very real concerns, and in no way is this book intended as a judgment on those who don't have the means or access to these luxuries.

The reality, however, is that the industrial food chain is making people very sick. Eric Schlosser, author of *Fast Food Nation,*[8] sums it up nicely in an editorial he penned for the *Washington Post* in 2011. In reference to the exotic ingredients and expensive meals championed by prominent foodies he writes, "Those things may be irritating. But they generally don't sicken or kill people. And our current industrial food system does."[9] We all have a stake in making our food safer and healthier for ourselves and our children, but change can only occur if those of us who do have the time and willingness to think about these things actually do something about it.

The food system in the United States is dominated by politics and a handful of corporations* that have a very strong interest in maintaining the status quo. These forces work to artificially deflate the price of industrial food with large government subsidies, while artificially inflating the price of smaller-scale food production with incongruent safety regulations.[10] The apparent elitism of high-priced, difficult to attain, organic grass-fed beef, for example, is really an artifact of a system that favors industrial food production over smaller, family-run farms. In countries where such policies do not exist (e.g., most of Europe), real food is considered normal, not elitist.

Modern agriculture has accomplished some amazing feats, and the goal is not to disregard these and move backward to a nonexistent era of pastoral bliss. There are still plenty of challenges to making sustainable, organic farming a viable option for feeding the nation, but our country has never been short on innovation. A new generation of young, enthusiastic farmers is pioneering new technologies and farming practices that make better food more affordable and easier to attain. It's really exciting to see, and I think future generations of foodists will look back at this time as the Renaissance of real food and sustainable agriculture.

Farmers markets and Whole Foods aren't in everyone's budget, but that doesn't mean that we should turn our backs on real food. As Eric Schlosser goes on to explain in his *Washington Post* piece, "The wealthy

---

*Props to them for convincing most of the country that small family farms are more elitist than their own multimillion-dollar operations.

will always eat well. It's the poor and working people who need a new, sustainable food system more than anyone else. They live in the most polluted neighborhoods. They are exposed to the worst toxic chemicals on the job. They are sold the unhealthiest foods and can least afford the medical problems that result." The popularizing of the food movement will inevitably lead to some extravagance—we all love to fantasize about once-in-a-lifetime, decadent meals. But it also raises awareness of the sometimes life-or-death issues that come with food production, which helps consumers make more informed choices and sways voters and politicians* to build a system that supports healthier food for everyone.

LIFE SHOULD BE AWESOME

At the end of the day, and at the end of your life, the reasons you choose for eating well really don't matter. The results are all that count. Choosing real food over edible products puts you on a path toward better health, a slimmer body, and a richer, more fulfilling life than any dieter could dream of. You'll protect yourself and your family from the most common chronic diseases of our time, so you can live out your days active and involved in the world. Sacrifice and willpower will be eliminated from your weight-loss tool kit and be replaced by delicious food and mindfulness, enabling you to savor everything worth eating. Your weight will settle at a new set point, where you can maintain it comfortably, without stress.

It's not an easy journey, but upgrading your healthstyle isn't particularly difficult either. By far the hardest part is getting started, breaking free from the clutches of habit that have you convinced that buying vegetables, cooking dinner, or walking that extra flight of stairs is impossibly difficult, habits that make you think you need superhuman

---

*At least the ones who aren't in the pockets of food corporations.

strength of will and resolve to stop eating from the candy jar at the office. Your habits, in other words, are the only things holding you back from taking the first step toward your new life and new body.

Habits make change difficult, but they (and therefore the difficulty) only exist in your mind. You now have a blueprint for rescripting old habits, so that your daily routines work for you instead of against you. You know how to turn healthy eating from a punishment into something you adore. You know how to recognize when less is more and how to optimize your food choices for health and pleasure. You know how to eat like a foodist.

ACKNOWLEDGMENTS

Foodist would still be a twinkle in my eye if it weren't for all the amazing people who have supported me throughout my career. First and foremost I'd like to thank my readers, whose endless feedback and encouragement have helped me refine my ideas and turn Summer Tomato into the tremendous resource it has become. I am constantly amazed by the high level of thought, dialogue, and compassion you have shown to one another and to me, and this book would not exist without you. Thank you deeply.

Special thanks to Patrick Birke, Cheryl-Ann Roberge, Kevin Systrom, Shayne Sweeney, Adam Gazzaley, and Michael Dempsey for allowing me to share your stories. You are inspirations to us all.

No individual has provided more physical and emotional support than my amazing husband, Kevin Rose. Thank you, love, for giving me the ability to follow my dreams, and for always knowing when I need help with dinner or a trip to a warm beach. I also need to thank our adorable labradoodle, Toaster, for making sure that no matter how much work needs to be done, there's always time to go for a walk.

I'm still astounded that my agent, Lisa DiMona, was courting me to represent this book, instead of the other way around. Lisa, you're a total rockstar. Thank you for believing in me before I had a fancy endorsement from *TIME*. I'll never forget that.

Huge thanks to the entire team at HarperOne, especially Mark Tauber and my editor, Gideon Weil. Somehow I doubt publishing is always this easy, but you guys made it feel like a summer breeze. Thank you for understanding my vision from the beginning and for helping me see it through. I am incredibly grateful for all your wisdom and support.

Thanks also to Suzanne Quist and Babette Dunkelgrun for your tremendous help and enthusiasm.

Thank you, Sam Wilson, for your encouragement, vigilant editing, and the *Twin Peaks* soundtrack that got me through this book. You were the first to explain to me the difference between a good sentence and a crappy one, and for that I'm eternally grateful.

I am incredibly fortunate to have a dream team of friends and mentors who have been willing to donate their time and wisdom to helping a youngling find her way in the big world of publishing. I'd especially like to thank Michael Pollan for encouraging me to "just start writing," when starting a new career felt even scarier than continuing an unsatisfying one.

A million thank-yous to Tim Ferriss for countless conversations about writing, publishing, marketing, blogging, eating, traveling, and everything in between. Tim's first book, *The 4-Hour Workweek,* is also what enabled me to launch a writing career while simultaneously finishing my Ph.D. I am forever in your debt, good sir.

No one has been as instrumental in my career and development as an individual as my dear friend and colleague Adam Gazzaley. Thanks, Adam, for giving me a chance when no one else would and for being a dedicated foodist guinea pig. I don't know where I would have been without your advice and support over the years. I look forward to many more workouts, conversations, and good times, because all of life is a celebration of life.

Thanks to Andrea Clements, Cheryl Clements, and David Goodman, for nearly three decades of love and support, and for helping me to grow into the person I am today. It's because of you three that I can instantly recognize a true friend when I see one.

Finally, I want to thank my dad, Michael. Dad, since before I can remember, you've always been my number one fan. You have more capacity for love, honesty, and selflessness than any person I've ever met, and you continue to be my inspiration and guiding light. I love you with all my heart. Thank you for everything.

NOTES

One: "Diet" Is a Four-Letter Word

1. Michael Pollan, "Our National Eating Disorder," *New York Times Magazine,* October 17, 2004.
2. Traci Mann et al., "Medicare's Search for Effective Obesity Treatments: Diets Are Not the Answer," *American Psychologist* 62, no. 3 (April 2007): 220–33.
3. Michael Pollan, *In Defense of Food* (New York: Penguin, 2008).

Two: The Myth of Willpower

1. If you need convincing, read Baumeister and Tierney's *Willpower: Rediscovering the Greatest Human Strength* (New York: Penguin, 2011) or read up on David Blaine (e.g., http://en.wikipedia.org/wiki/David_Blaine).
2. Baumeister and Tierney, *Willpower,* p. 217.
3. M. T. Gailliot et al., "Self-control Relies on Glucose as a Limited Energy Source: Willpower Is More Than a Metaphor," *Journal of Personality and Social Psychology* 92, no. 2 (February 2007): 325–36.
4. Baumeister and Tierney, *Willpower,* p. 150.
5. Denise T. de Ridder et al., "Taking Stock of Self-Control: A Meta-Analysis of How Trait Self-Control Relates to a Wide Range of Behaviors," *Personality and Social Psychology Review* 16, no. 1 (February 2012): 76–99.
6. Michael Pollan, *The Omnivore's Dilemma* (New York: Penguin, 2006).
7. De Ridder et al., "Taking Stock of Self-Control," p. 79.
8. Carol S. Dweck, *Mindset: The New Psychology of Success* (New York: Ballantine, 2006).

Three: Healthstyle

1. Personal e-mail interview with Nicole Mead, March 29, 2012.
2. Chip Heath and Dan Heath, *Switch: How to Change Things When Change Is Hard* (New York: Crown, 2010).
3. Brian Wansink, *Mindless Eating: Why We Eat More Than We Think* (New York: Bantam, 2006).
4. Charles Duhigg, *The Power of Habit* (New York: Random House, 2012).

5. David T. Neal et al., "The Pull of the Past: When Do Habits Persist Despite Conflict with Motives?" *Personality and Social Psychology Bulletin* 37, no. 11 (November 2011): 1428–37.

Four: Eat Food

1. For an excellent review, I highly recommend Michael Pollan, *In Defense of Food* (New York: Penguin, 2008).
2. Michael Chu and Terry F. Seltzer, "Letter to the Editor: Myxedema Coma Induced by Ingestion of Raw Bok Choy," *New England Journal of Medicine* 362 (May 20, 2010): 1945–46.
3. http://www.montereybayaquarium.org/cr/seafoodwatch.aspx.
4. http://www.montereybayaquarium.org/cr/cr_seafoodwatch/sfw_health.aspx.
5. Arne Astrup et al., "The Role of Reducing Intakes of Saturated Fat in the Prevention of Cardiovascular Disease: Where Does the Evidence Stand in 2010?" *American Journal of Clinical Nutrition* 93, no. 4 (April 2011): 684–88.
6. Timothy Ferriss, *The 4-Hour Body* (New York: Crown, 2010).
7. I. Björck et al., "Food Properties Affecting the Digestion and Absorption of Carbohydrates," *American Journal of Clinical Nutrition* 59, no. 3 Suppl. (March 1994): 699S–705S.
8. N. Tsukahara and I. Ezawa, "Calcium Intake and Osteoporosis in Many Countries," *Clinical Calcium* 11, no. 2 (February 2001): 173–77.
9. C. A. Gonzalez and E. Riboli, "Diet and Cancer Prevention," *European Journal of Cancer* 46, no. 14 (September 2010): 2555–62.
10. I. R. Reid, M. J. Bolland, and A. Grey, "Effect of Calcium Supplementation on Hip Fractures," *Osteoporosis International* 19, no. 8 (August 2008): 1119–23.
11. B. M. Tang et al., "Use of Calcium or Calcium in Combination with Vitamin D Supplementation to Prevent Fractures and Bone Loss in People Aged 50 Years and Older: A Meta-analysis," *Lancet* 370, no. 9588 (August 25, 2007): 657–66.
12. Y. Park et al., "Dairy Food, Calcium, and Risk of Cancer in the NIH-AARP Diet and Health Study," *Archives of Internal Medicine* 169, no. 4 (February 23, 2009): 391–401.
13. P. J. Huth and K. M. Park, "Influence of Dairy Product and Milk Fat Consumption on Cardiovascular Disease Risk: A Review of the Evidence," *Advanced Nutrition* 3, no. 3 (May 1, 2012): 266–85; doi: 10.3945/an.112.002030.
14. J. M. Geleijnse et al., "Dietary Intake of Menaquinone Is Associated with a Reduced Risk of Coronary Heart Disease: The Rotterdam Study," *Journal of Nutrition* 134, no. 11 (November 2004): 3100–105.
15. G. C. Gast et al., "A High Menaquinone Intake Reduces the Incidence of Coronary Heart Disease," *Nutrition, Metabolism, and Cardiovascular Diseases* 19, no. 7 (September 2009): 504–10.
16. K. Nimptsch et al., "Dietary Vitamin K Intake in Relation to Cancer Incidence and Mortality," *American Journal of Clinical Nutrition* 91, no. 5 (May 2010): 1348–58.
17. F. Fumeron et al., "Dairy Consumption and the Incidence of Hyperglycemia and the Metabolic Syndrome," *Diabetes Care* 34, no. 4 (April 2011): 813–17.

18. L. Duedahl-Olesen et al., "Influence of Smoking Parameters on the Concentration of Polycyclic Aromatic Hydrocarbons (PAHs) in Danish Smoked Fish," *Food Additives & Contaminants: Part A, Chemistry, Analysis, Control, Exposure, and Risk Assessment* 27, no. 9 (September 2010): 1294–305.

19. José M. Lorenzo et al., "Polycyclic Aromatic Hydrocarbons (PAHs) in Two Spanish Traditional Smoked Sausage Varieties: 'Androlla' and 'Bolillo,'" *Meat Science* 86, no. 3 (November 2010): 660–64; "Polycyclic Aromatic Hydrocarbons (PAHs) in Two Spanish Traditional Smoked Sausage Varieties: 'Chorizo gallego' and 'Chorizo de cebolla,'" *Meat Science* 89, no. 1 (September 2011): 105–9; C. Santos, A. Gomes, and L. C. Roseiro, "Polycyclic Aromatic Hydrocarbons Incidence in Portuguese Traditional Smoked Meat Products," *Food and Chemical Toxicology* 49, no. 9 (September 2011): 2343–47.

20. Pollan, *In Defense of Food,* p. 1.

Five: Know Thy Food

1. Brian Wansink and Pierre Chandon, "Meal Size, Not Body Size, Explains Errors in Estimating the Calorie Content of Meals," *Annals of Internal Medicine* 145, no. 5 (September 2006): 326–32.

2. Ruth Reichl, *Garlic and Sapphires* (New York: Penguin, 2005).

Six: Shopping and Cooking

1. Jake Claro, "Vermont Farmers Markets and Grocery Stores: A Price Comparison," http://nofavt.org/sites/default/files/NOFA%20Price%20Study.pdf.

Seven: Zen and the Art of Mindful Eating

1. S. Tanihara et al., "Retrospective Longitudinal Study on the Relationship Between 8-Year Weight Change and Current Eating Speed, *Appetite* 57, no. 1 (August 2011): 179–83.

2. J. Galhardo et al., "Normalizing Eating Behavior Reduces Body Weight and Improves Gastrointestinal Hormonal Secretion in Obese Adolescents," *Journal of Clinical Endocrinology & Metabolism* 97, no. 2 (February 2012): E193–201.

3. Malcolm Gladwell, *Blink: The Power of Thinking Without Thinking* (New York: Little, Brown, 2005).

Eight: The Way You Move

1. M. S. Tremblay et al., "Physiological and Health Implications of a Sedentary Lifestyle," *Applied Physiology, Nutrition, and Metabolism* 35, no. 6 (December 2010): 725–40.

2. A. J. Levine, "Nonexercise Activity Thermogenesis (NEAT): Environment and Biology," *American Journal of Physiology: Endocrinology and Metabolism* 286, no. 5 (May 2004): E675–85.

3. M. A. Alahmadi et al., "Exercise Intensity Influences Nonexercise Activity Thermogenesis in Overweight and Obese Adults," *Medicine and Science in Sports and Exercise* 43, no. 4 (April 2011): 624–31.

Nine: Recalibration, Troubleshooting, and Maintenance

1. USDA, Agriculture Fact Book, 2001–2002 (chapter 2), "Profiling Food Consumption in America," www.usda.gov/factbook.
2. Stephan Guyenet, Whole Health Source: Ancestral Nutrition and Health, http://wholehealthsource.blogspot.com.
3. Stephan Guyenet, Whole Health Source: Ancestral Nutrition and Health, http://wholehealthsource.blogspot.com.
4. Stephan Guyenet, "By 2606, the US Diet Will Be 100 Percent Sugar," http://whole healthsource.blogspot.com, February 18, 2012.
5. D. Thomas and E. J. Elliott, "Low Glycaemic Index, or Low Glycaemic Load, Diets for Diabetes Mellitus," *Cochrane Database of Systematic Reviews* 1 (January 21, 2009): CD006296.
6. J. L. Fortuna, "Sweet Preference, Sugar Addiction and the Familial History of Alcohol Dependence: Shared Neural Pathways and Genes," *Journal of Psychoactive Drugs* 42, no. 2 (June 2010): 147–51.
7. A. Salehi et al., "The Insulinogenic Effect of Whey Protein Is Partially Mediated by a Direct Effect of Amino Acids and GIP on [beta symbol]-cells," *Nutrition and Metabolism (London)* 9, no. 1 (May 30, 2012): 48; doi: 10.1186/1743-7075-9-48.
8. E. H. Spencer, H. R. Ferdowsian, and N. D. Barbard, "Diet and Acne: A Review of the Evidence," *International Journal of Dermatology* 48, no. 4 (April 2009): 339–47.
9. N. S. Scrimshaw and E. B. Murray, "The Acceptability of Milk and Milk Products in Populations with a High Prevalence of Lactose Intolerance," *American Journal of Clinical Nutrition* 48, supp. 4 (October 1988): 1079–159. T. Sahi, "Genetics and Epidemiology of Adult-Type Hypolactasia," *Scandinavian Journal of Gastroenterology,* suppl. 202 (1994): 7–20. E. Gudmand-Høyer, "The Clinical Significance of Disaccharide Maldigestion," *American Journal of Clinical Nutrition* 9, suppl. 3 (March 1994): 7353–415.
10. E. B. Rimm et al., "Moderate Alcohol Intake and Lower Risk of Coronary Heart Disease: Meta-Analysis of Effects on Lipids and Haemostatic Factors," *British Medical Journal* 319, no. 7224 (December 11, 1999): 1523–28.
11. S. C. Larrson, E. Giovannucci, and A. Wolk, "Folate and Risk of Breast Cancer: A Meta-Analysis," *National Cancer Institute* 99, no. 1 (January 3, 2007): 64–76.
12. D. E. Thomas, E. J. Elliott, and G. A. Naughton, "Exercise for Type 2 Diabetes Mellitus," *Cochrane Database of Systematic Reviews* 3 (July 19, 2006): CD002968.
13. Richard E. Keesey and Matt D. Hirvonen, "Body Weight Set-Points: Determination and Adjustment," *Journal of Nutrition* 127, no. 9 (September 1, 1997): 1875S–83S.

Ten: Home Savory Home

1. A. G. Liu et al., "Reducing the Glycemic Index or Carbohydrate Content of Mixed Meals Reduces Postprandial Glycemia and Insulinemia Over the Entire Day but Does Not Affect Satiety," *Diabetes Care* 35, no. 8 (August 2012): 1633–37.
2. G. S. Masterton and P. C. Hayes, "Coffee and the Liver: A Potential Treatment for Liver Disease?" *European Journal of Gastroenterology and Hepatology* 22, no. 11 (November 2010): 1277–83.
3. L. Arab, "Epidemiologic Evidence on Coffee and Cancer," *Nutrition and Cancer* 62, no. 3 (2010): 271–83.
4. R. Huxley et al., "Coffee, Decaffeinated Coffee, and Tea Consumption in Relation to Incident Type 2 Diabetes Mellitus: A Systematic Review with Meta-Analysis," *Archives of Internal Medicine* 169, no. 22 (December 14, 2009): 2053–63.
5. G. W. Arendash and C. Cao, "Caffeine and Coffee as Therapeutics Against Alzheimer's Disease," *Journal of Alzheimer's Disease* 20, suppl. 1 (2010): S117–26.
6. J. Costa et al., "Caffeine Exposure and the Risk of Parkinson's Disease: A Systematic Review and Meta-Analysis of Observational Studies," *Journal of Alzheimer's Disease* 20, suppl. 1 (2010): S221–38.
7. C. Santos et al., "Caffeine Intake and Dementia: Systematic Review and Meta-Analysis," *Journal of Alzheimer's Disease* 20, suppl. 1 (2010): S187–204.
8. T. A. Astorino and D. W. Robertson, "Efficacy of Acute Caffeine Ingestion for Short-Term High-Intensity Exercise Performance: A Systematic Review," *Journal of Strength and Conditioning Research* 24, no. 1 (January 2010): 257–65.
9. A. E. Mesas et al., "The Effect of Coffee on Blood Pressure and Cardiovascular Disease in Hypertensive Individuals: A Systematic Review and Meta-analysis," *American Journal of Clinical Nutrition* 94, no. 4 (October 2011): 1113–26.
10. J. M. Geleijnse, "Habitual Coffee Consumption and Blood Pressure: An Epidemiological Perspective," *Journal of Vascular Health and Risk Management* 4, no. 5 (2008): 963–70.
11. A. C. Grandjean et al., "The Effect of Caffeinated, Non-Caffeinated, Caloric and Non-Caloric Beverages on Hydration," *Journal of the American College of Nutrition* 19, no. 5 (October 2000): 591–600.

Eleven: The Office

1. Vanessa M. Patrick and Henrik Hagtvedt, "Empowered Refusal Motivates Goal-Directed Behavior," *Journal of Consumer Research* 39, no. 2 (August 2010): 371–81.
2. Tim Ferriss, *The 4-Hour Chef* (New York: Houghton Mifflin Harcourt, 2012).

Thirteen: How to Win Over Friends and Influence Family

1. Brian Wansink, *Marketing Nutrition* (Urbana: Univ. of Illinois Press, 2005), p. 38.
2. Wansink, *Marketing Nutrition,* p. 38.
3. Wansink, *Marketing Nutrition,* p. 39.

4. Pierre Chandon and Brian Wansink, "The Biasing Health Halos of Fast-Food Restaurant Health Claims: Lower Calorie Estimates and Higher Side-Dish Consumption Intentions," *Journal of Consumer Research* 34, no. 3 (October 2007): 301–14.

5. Wansink, *Marketing Nutrition,* pp. 35–36.

6. Wansink, *Marketing Nutrition,* p. 41.

7. S. Y. Lee, S. L. Hoerr, and R. F. Schiffman, "Screening for Infants' and Toddlers' Dietary Quality Through Maternal Diet," *MCN, American Journal of Maternal/Child Nursing* 30, no. 1 (January–February 2005): 60–66.

8. F. Zampollo, K. M. Kniffin, B. Wansink, and M. Shimizu, "Food Plating Preferences of Children: The Importance of Presentation on Desire for Diversity," *Acta Paediatrica* 101, no. 1 (January 2012): 61–66.

9. A. Remington et al., "Increasing Food Acceptance in the Home Setting: A Randomized Controlled Trial of Parent-Administered Taste Exposure with Incentives," *American Journal of Clinical Nutrition* 95, no. 1 (January 2012): 72–77.

10. K. van der Horst, "Overcoming Picky Eating: Eating Enjoyment as a Central Aspect of Children's Eating Behaviors," *Appetite* 58, no. 2 (April 2012): 567–74.

11. I. J. Brown et al., "Salt Intakes Around the World: Implications for Public Health," *International Journal of Epidemiology* 38, no. 3 (June 2009): 791–813.

12. M. Camões et al., "The Role of Physical Activity and Diet in the Incidence of Hypertension: A Population-Based Study in Portuguese Adults," *European Journal of Clinical Nutrition* 64, no. 12 (December 2010): 1441–49.

13. M. Madero et al., "Dietary Fructose and Hypertension," *Current Hypertension Reports* 13, no. 1 (February 2011): 29–35.

Fourteen: On Food and Values

1. E. B. Hekler, C. D. Gardner, and T. N. Robinson, "Effects of a College Course About Food and Society on Students' Eating Behaviors," *American Journal of Preventative Medicine* 38, no. 5 (May 2010): 543–47.

2. Joel Salatin, *Folks, This Ain't Normal* (New York: Center Street, 2011).

3. Jeff Benedict, *Poisoned* (Buena Vista, VA: Inspire Books, 2011).

4. Barry Estabrook, *Tomatoland* (Kansas City, MO: Andrews McMeel, 2011).

5. A. Oppliger, "Antimicrobial Resistance of Staphylococcus Aureus Strains Acquired by Pig Farmers from Pigs," *Applied and Environmental Microbiology* 78, no. 22 (November 2012): 8010–14; L. B. Price et al., "Staphylococcus Aureus CC398: Host Adaptation and Emergence of Methicillin Resistance in Livestock," *mBio* 3, no. 1 (February 2012): pii: e00305–11; doi: 10.1128/mBio.00305–11.

6. M. F. K. Fisher, *The Art of Eating* (Hoboken: Wiley, 2004), p. 353.

7. Michael Pollan, *The Omnivore's Dilemma* (New York: Penguin, 2006).

8. Eric Schlosser, *Fast Food Nation* (Boston: Houghton Mifflin, 2001).

9. Eric Schlosser, "Why Being a Foodie Isn't 'Elitist,' " http://www.washingtonpost.com/opinions/why-being-a-foodie-isnt-elitist/2011/04/27/AFeWsnFF_story.html.

10. Read Joel Salatin's, *Everything I Want to Do Is Illegal: War Stories from the Local Food Front* (Swoope, VA: Polyface, 2007) for more on this brand of ridiculousness.

INDEX

saturated fat from, 186
serving size, 69n
meat substitutes, 60
metabolic syndrome, 17–18, 75, 188
metabolism
   breakfast and, 211
   dieting and slowing of, 198, 201
   factors in, 55, 55n
   insulin resistance and, 186, 249
   returning to normal, 188–89
   set point, 198–99
micronutrients, 55, 58
mindful eating, 22–23, 95, 149–172, 197
   breaking the fast eating habit, 152–58
   18 tips to eat more slowly and mindfully,
     154–58
   restaurant meals and, 273
Mindless Eating (Wansink), 40, 281
mindset, 26–27, 50–51
Mindset (Dweck), 26–27
mint: Roasted Beets with Fresh Mint and
   Chèvre, 294–95
mobile apps, 93, 111n
monitoring food intake, 91–113, 206
   identifying rewards, 99–101
   journaling, 92–98
   looking for triggers, 98–99
   mobile apps for, 93
   sample foodist's journal, 96–98
   taking inventory, 101–2
   weighing yourself and, 110–12
Monterey Bay Aquarium's lists, 64, 65
muesli, 103, 211
mushrooms, 72, 132–33

NEAT, 109, 174–78, 179, 196
niacin, 69
Nike+ FuelBand, 109n, 256
Norris, Kathleen, 115
nuts, 130, 158, 232
   Pan-Roasted Brussels Sprouts with Bacon,
     167–68
   Sautéed Kale with Pistachios and Garlic,
     239–40
   toasting, 167

oats, 192n, 194
obesity, 140, 152, 187
oligosaccharides, 219, 220, 223, 225, 226
olive oil, 68, 127

olives, 134
omega-3 fatty acids, 62, 66, 66n, 68
Omnivore's Dilemma, The (Pollan), 5, 24,
   309
onions, small, 135
organic foods, 18, 87, 137, 138, 142, 147,
   195, 264, 286, 307, 309, 310
osteoporosis, 75
overeating, 149–52
oysters, 70, 73

padróns, 292
Painter, James, 151
parsley, 136
pasta, servings per week, 74
Patrick, Vanessa, 36–37, 247
Pavarotti, Luciano, 265
pepper (peppercorns), 128
phytic acid, 73–74
picky eaters, 171
   foodists vs., 172
   food texture and, 167–72
   "Gateway Vegetables" story, 163–65
   taste and, 162–67
pistachio nuts: Sautéed Kale with Pistachios
   and Garlic, 239–40
plastic items, 222
   bisphenol A (BPA) in, 130
   bowls, 123
   cutting boards, 122, 122n
   storage containers, 127, 222n
Pleasure, Samuel, 35n
Poisoned (Benedict), 306
Pollan, Michael, 5, 7, 12, 24, 53, 83, 309
portion size, 9, 22, 41, 74, 92–93, 95, 151–52,
   157
   meats, 69n
   plate, glass, or utensil size and, 40, 41
   restaurant meals, 266–67
Portion Size Me (film), 151–52
potassium, 297
potatoes, 72, 274
Power of Habit, The (Duhigg, Charles), 45
prediabetes, 188, 296
probiotics, 224
processed foods, 56–57, 68, 83, 84, 87
   diabetes and, 249, 296
   diseases of civilization and, 248–49
   meats, 68, 82–83, 82n
   salt intake and, 127, 297–98

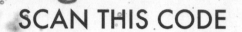

SCAN THIS CODE
WITH YOUR SMARTPHONE TO BE LINKED TO
THE BONUS MATERIALS FOR

FOODIST

on the Elixir mobile website,
where you can also find information about other
healthy living books and related materials.

YOU CAN ALSO TEXT
FOODIST to READIT (732348)

to be sent a link to the Elixir mobile website.